"*Relax into Yoga for Chronic Pain* is the rare resource that combines insights from modern neuroscience and psychology, wisdom from long-practiced healing traditions, and tremendous compassion for the experience of living with chronic pain. I highly recommend this book and the practices in it."

—**Kelly McGonigal, PhD**, author of *Yoga for Pain Relief*

"Einstein defined genius as making the complex simple. *Relax into Yoga for Chronic Pain* is genius. This book is so accessible with simple, powerful practices for the reader while still conveying the depth and complexity of our best understanding of pain. The weaving together of the information, activities, and reflection exercises offers safe, comprehensive, and appropriate support for those living with persistent pain. The book would also make an outstanding student workbook for yoga teachers and therapists to offer eight-week training programs in their community. The reader will enjoy and benefit from 'riding the wave' of this masterful guidebook."

—**Matthew J. Taylor, PT, PhD, C-IAYT**, director of SmartSafeYoga, national yoga safety expert, and author of *Yoga Therapy as a Creative Response to Pain*

"This book is a gem! Easily understandable in its text, illustrations, and guided meditations, this is an excellent choice that is likely to inform and help anyone living with chronic pain. The authors have many years of dedicated personal practice experience with both mindfulness and yoga. In addition, they have extensive experience teaching and training others to use these approaches in the service of better health and more effective management of serious medical conditions like chronic pain. Their expertise, dedication, and beautiful compassion shine throughout this work!"

—**Jeffrey Brantley, MD**, founding faculty member at Duke Integrative Medicine; assistant consulting professor in the department of psychiatry and behavioral sciences at Duke University Medical Center; author of *Calming Your Anxious Mind*; and coauthor of the *Five Good Minutes* series

"This book is a standout among yoga guides. It is supported by both empiric scientific data and Jim Carson's experience living in India as a monk in the yoga tradition. This truly unique guide to reclaiming yourself through mindful yoga is life-changing. Learn to 'ride the waves' and start enjoying your life again, today."

—**Kim Dupree Jones, PhD, RN, FAAN**, professor and dean of Linfield School of Nursing; research faculty at Oregon Health and Science University; and chronic pain researcher who has produced over 400 peer-reviewed papers, presentations, and chapters, and has been supported by federal, foundation, and industry funders

"Well paced, *Relax into Yoga for Chronic Pain* expands yoga from body movements to a variety of skills for deepening awareness of how one relates to unwanted experience. This down-to-earth guide is filled with compassion and wisdom as it empowers learning and practice, reflection, and engagement to 'ride the waves' of strong sensations, challenging emotions, and constricting thoughts that tangle together with chronic pain. Through acknowledgement of the innate resource of presence, patience and love can flourish. This book has the potential to support working with pain in practical ways that support the emergence of greater peace, energy, and joy."

—**Florence Meleo-Meyer, MS, MA**, program director for the Global Relations and Professional Education Mindfulness Center at the Brown University School of Public Health

"When pain persists, access to effective, evidence-based care is vital. The right guidance is equally important to finding and practicing individualized solutions. *Relax into Yoga for Chronic Pain* is a practical coaching tool—building understanding, a repertoire of techniques, and self-assessment expertise in an eight-week program that demonstrates our ability to influence pain, fatigue, sleep, mood, and ease of movement. This is an excellent integration of science and yoga that will provide relief to many people living in pain."

—**Neil Pearson, PT, MSc (RHBS), BA-BPHE, CIAYT, ERYT500**, clinical assistant professor at the University of British Columbia, physical therapist, yoga therapist, and author/coeditor of *Yoga and Science in Pain Care*

"This wonderful instruction manual is just what the doctor ordered! As physicians, we often tell patients suffering from chronic pain that yoga and meditation will help, but classes can be overwhelming or intimidating. Finally, here is a workbook that guides the reader through simple exercises and movements while explaining how yoga philosophy and practice can change our perception of chronic pain."

    —**Kimberly Mauer, MD**, director of the Comprehensive Pain Management Center, and clinical associate professor of anesthesiology and perioperative medicine at Oregon Health and Science University

"*Relax into Yoga for Chronic Pain* offers real-world solutions for people who may not have the strength, stamina, or flexibility to do the kinds of acrobatic yoga you see in magazines and on social media. This is yoga that meets you where you are, and gradually builds from there. Even a few minutes per day of the poses, breathing exercises, relaxation techniques, and other yoga practices skillfully described in this book could make an enormous difference not just in your pain, but in your whole life."

    —**Timothy McCall, MD**, author of *Yoga as Medicine* and *Saving My Neck*, and medical editor for *Yoga Journal*

Relax into Yoga *for* Chronic Pain

An Eight-Week
Mindful Yoga Workbook
for Finding Relief
and Resilience

JIM CARSON, PhD

KIMBERLY CARSON, MPH, C-IAYT

CAROL KRUCOFF, C-IAYT

New Harbinger Publications, Inc.

Publisher's Note

This publication is designed to provide accurate and authoritative information in regard to the subject matter covered. It is sold with the understanding that the publisher is not engaged in rendering psychological, financial, legal, or other professional services. If expert assistance or counseling is needed, the services of a competent professional should be sought.

Distributed in Canada by Raincoast Books

Copyright © 2019 by Jim Carson, Kimberly Carson, and Carol Krucoff
        New Harbinger Publications, Inc.
        5674 Shattuck Avenue
        Oakland, CA 94609
        www.newharbinger.com

Cover design by Amy Daniel

Acquired by Jess O'Brien

Edited by Marisa Solís

Library of Congress Cataloging-in-Publication Data on file

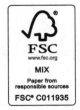
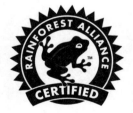

Printed in the United States of America

21   20   19

10 9 8 7 6 5 4 3 2 1   First Printing

"The heart is the hub of all sacred places. Go there and roam."

—Bhagawan Nityananda

Contents

FOREWORD

Yoga Can Help

As I write these words, before this book is even published, it already feels indispensable. Yoga has become more popular than ever in recent years—available in virtually every health club in the United States and beyond, inspiring lifestyle brands that have become big business. Yet even as it becomes more ubiquitous, finding yoga classes well suited to individuals with chronic pain remains challenging.

This workbook and the practices it sets out through its eight-week Mindful Yoga program, along with the links to online audio and video resources to further support learning the yoga skills it introduces, fills this gap. *Relax into Yoga for Chronic Pain* skillfully interweaves the latest scientific information on the biological, psychological, and lifestyle factors that contribute to chronic pain, with clear descriptions of yoga-based tools and their recommended uses to effectively manage pain.

Most important, this book will support you in being able to return to the activities that make life meaningful to you—activities that many people with chronic pain gave up on long ago. Interspersed throughout the book are inspiring stories that bring to life how others, debilitated by pain and discouraged beyond action, found a path back to a full and meaningful life through the yoga-based practices that Kimberly Carson, Jim Carson, and Carol Krucoff carefully lay out.

Kimberly worked closely with me and my research team to bring many of these practices to hundreds of members of the Kaiser Permanente health care systems in Georgia, Hawaii, and the Pacific Northwest. I've witnessed firsthand the remarkable difference these practices made in many of these individuals' lives, all of whom were on long-term opioids for their chronic pain. These practices were essential in giving them a way of getting back in the driver's seat in leading their day-to-day lives, without relying on a medication that we now know can lead to more problems over time, yet would never provide the transformative change that these yoga-based tools and similar lifestyle approaches make possible.

This program makes yoga accessible to everyone by encouraging you to start where you're at—practicing the physical poses in and with the support of a chair, and progressing to a floor-based practice when and if this makes sense for you. Yet as important as these physical practices can be in restoring functioning and confidence for those who have often been compromised by their chronic pain, the program in this book goes far beyond the physical practice of yoga.

In recent years, the critical connections between our thinking (that is, the stories we tell ourselves), our attentional focus, our emotional experience, and why and how extensively we experience pain has been made startling clear by new research. The authors do a skillful job of bringing their wisdom and deep experience to this larger focus by easing the reader into the holistic yogic practices of meditation, breathing exercises, and self-study. In so doing, they present a comprehensive program that, from a yogic perspective, addresses many of the key tenets of cognitive-behavioral therapies.

Fully following the path set forth in this program can enable a fundamental shift in your relationship to pain, removing it from center stage and promoting deep healing. While I have utmost confidence that such a transformation is probable if you faithfully follow the steps outlined in these chapters, each chapter also anticipates the inevitable challenges that most people face in trying to embed these practices into their day-to-day lives. The authors review how to overcome such obstacles with curiosity and compassion toward oneself, while steering clear of the all-too-common toughen-up or "pull oneself up by the bootstraps" mentality that often fails to lead to enduring behavior change.

This book is beautifully written and a pleasure to read. It very intentionally builds on a central metaphor—that of riding, not battling, the waves of attention, stress, the mind's story, pain, emotion, and fatigue—the many challenges that inevitably accompany one on the journey with chronic pain. This book will guide you in gently navigating these challenges.

Most helpful, it cuts through the scientific jargon that can contribute to a stigmatization and feeling of responsibility for one's pain that is so disappointingly pervasive in our health care systems. I expect this book and the program it describes will become an increasingly common foundation for the best available care for chronic pain.

That said, taking advantage of this approach doesn't require being guided by a health care practitioner—the book and the online resources it provides are complete unto themselves. Read it, live it, practice what is presented in this program and you're in for a remarkable and life-transforming journey. Enjoy!

—Lynn DeBar, PhD
Senior Investigator, Kaiser Permanente Washington Health Research
Institute, Seattle, Washington

INTRODUCTION

What Is Chronic Pain and How Can Mindful Yoga Help?

The practice of yoga relies on these foundations:
Forbearance in the face of difficulties,
The pursuit of self-knowledge, and
Receptivity to pure awareness.
Yoga's goals are to disarm the causes of suffering, and
reveal deep joy, peace, and clarity.

—Yoga Sutras of Patanjali

Quite likely, you are struggling with pain that seems to have sucked all the joy from your life. You're not sleeping, you've quit activities that you loved. You feel as if your pain is an anchor you have to drag around, and some days the anchor is so heavy that you can't perform the simplest tasks. We know. Because we work every day with people just like you, people who have tried everything with little success. Many came to mindfulness and yoga as a last resort. Now these former skeptics have become our biggest cheerleaders. Because our program works. And it can work for you too.

Pain is an inevitable part of being human. But in our stressful modern world, the chronic pain that you and millions of others feel has become an epidemic. One in three adults in the United States—more than 116 million people—experience chronic pain, a number that exceeds those affected by heart disease, cancer, and diabetes combined (Institute of Medicine 2011; Tsang et al. 2008). Pain is the primary reason people seek medical care. Beyond the suffering of individuals and families, chronic pain costs our country a staggering $635 billion each year in medical treatment and lost productivity (Institute of Medicine 2011). And it's not just an American problem. At any given time, about 20 percent of the worldwide population is experiencing chronic pain (Goldberg and McGee 2011).

You may have direct experience with the unfortunate reality that medications prescribed for pain have limited effectiveness and are often accompanied by harmful side effects (Martell et al. 2007; Russell et al. 2008). Tragically, more than 115 Americans die *every day* from overdosing on opioids, making drug overdose the leading cause of death for Americans under age fifty (National Institute on Drug Abuse 2018). As a result, *chronic pain and the opioid epidemic have been declared a public health crisis in America.*

Nationally, there is a growing urgency regarding the problem of dependence on opioid medications for chronic pain. Major health care organizations have issued guidelines for treating pain that recommend nondrug approaches—such as yoga and meditation—as the first line of treatment for chronic pain. While this shift to starting treatment with non-pharmacological approaches rather than powerful pills is healthy and commendable, it has also made it more difficult for those suffering from chronic pain to receive prescriptions for opioid medications. This has left countless Americans and their health care providers—who formerly relied on these drugs to relieve life-altering pain—with few options. Many of us are asking the question, "Now what?"

The harsh reality is that chronic pain is a complex phenomenon that is extremely difficult to manage well. In the past, providers had little to offer patients other than medication. But as experts in yoga and meditation, we the authors know these disciplines include powerful techniques that promise profound relief for people suffering from chronic pain (Villemure and Bushnell 2002). Inspired by the work of Jon Kabat-Zinn (1990), in 2000 Jim and Kimberly Carson began developing their Mindful Yoga program at Duke University Medical Center and testing its effects on people with varied kinds of chronic pain, including fibromyalgia, low-back pain, and cancer pain. Carol Krucoff joined them in this work a decade ago.

Today, the Carsons' substantial body of research shows that Mindful Yoga significantly reduces pain—and also relieves fatigue and emotional distress—*in some cases working more effectively than medication, and without negative side effects* (Carson et al. 2005, 2007, 2009, 2010, 2012, 2016). For more than twenty years, we've taught countless people how to use yoga and mindfulness strategies to reduce their pain levels and decrease their reliance on medications and medical procedures. *The results have often been dramatic*—for example, some people who needed strong drugs just to get out of bed in the morning were able to eliminate their need for prescription painkillers entirely. Others were able to resume their most cherished activities, like playing with the grandkids and camping in remote areas.

In general, most people who practice Mindful Yoga regularly find relief and are able to manage chronic pain with minimal pills. In addition, Mindful Yoga helps restore physical and emotional health, enhance vitality, and reclaim lives.

Right now, please take a few moments to reflect on what pain treatments you have tried. What therapies or strategies have worked best for you? What are your hopes for how this yoga program might help? Briefly summarize your experiences and hopes.

_____

_____

_____

_____

_____

Here's the story of one of Mindful Yoga's first participants, Debbie, who credits the practice with transforming her from being retired on disability to launching a successful second career.

Debbie's Story

Debbie's back pain started innocently enough when she was in her late thirties. A registered nurse, she "threw out her back" one day while lifting a patient onto a bed. After a few weeks, the sharp pain eased, but she continued to feel a nagging ache in her low back that never completely went away. With time, and the continued demands of her job, Debbie's backache got worse and made it increasingly difficult to do her job. She began experiencing pain in other parts of her body, and her doctor diagnosed her with fibromyalgia—a complex and poorly understood condition characterized by widespread chronic pain. In her early fifties, she was forced into retirement by a combination of fibromyalgia and low-back pain. Complicating Debbie's situation was her sense of persistent anxiety driven by memories of trauma she experienced growing up in an abusive home.

When Debbie first came to our Mindful Yoga program, she had been struggling to get more than a few hours of sleep most nights and was spending much of each day in bed. She despaired of no longer being able to care for her two horses that she loved dearly. At first, Debbie was afraid to try yoga for fear of getting hurt. Any attempt she'd made at exercising had ended in debilitating pain flares. As a result, she carried a great deal of tension in her muscles, which tended to grip in an effort to protect her back. Lack of activity had caused her to gain weight, which increased pressure on her knees and hips, and exacerbated her pain.

However, as she learned to move mindfully through gentle yoga postures, to observe internal patterns through daily meditation, and to work with her breath at intervals throughout the day,

Debbie found that her pain began to diminish. She arrived at class five of the eight-week course wearing a big smile. She said that while she was at the barn with her horses, she became aware of her mind's inner dialogue about how awful everything had become. As she noticed this thought pattern, she could sense how simultaneously her body tensed up and her pain increased. Rather than continue with that train of thought, Debbie redirected her attention to what she loved most— her horses. As she did, she felt her tension relax and her pain ease.

With this experience of working skillfully with her inner dynamics, Debbie said she "felt inspired for the first time in years!" Even her horses seemed to be able to tell the difference. She also found that the yogic approach of treating herself with compassion, and moving in ways that challenged but didn't strain her body, helped her more easily tolerate the discomfort that persisted.

Rather than lying awake in pain every night, Debbie began to sleep better, her energy improved, and her thoughts were no longer centered on a sense of distress. As she continued to feel and function better, her pain specialist told her that her progress was "astonishing" compared to her first visit several years before. In fact, her Manual Tender Point Survey score, which is used to diagnosis fibromyalgia, had dropped from the worst possible score, 18 out of 18, to only 6 out of 18.

Ultimately, Debbie entered a phase of new inspiration for her life and work. She'd always had artistic inclinations but never applied herself earnestly to artwork. But she soon discovered that she could produce award-winning sculptures and jewelry. These accomplishments launched her into a successful second career as the owner of a unique studio in the arts district of a major city. She told us that she feels very grateful for what she has gained from her yoga practices. She discovered that she could work with pain as a manageable challenge, rather than having it define and dominate her life.

The Perfect Storm of Chronic Pain

Debbie's case illustrates a chronic pain perfect storm that is similar to the experience of millions of people who suffer from this complex condition. Unlike acute pain, which occurs in response to an injury and then goes away, pain is considered "chronic" when it has persisted for three or more months (Institute of Medicine 2011).

Surprisingly, the mechanisms of chronic pain are quite different from how many people understand pain. Current neuroscience shows that *persistent pain actually rewires our brain*, so that the pain experience develops into a complex, self-sustaining neural network that is distinct from the original injury. Chronic pain involves much more than the actual damage in our body.

Despite the common belief that more pain means more damage, pain is frequently elevated by the thoughts, feelings, and other inputs we experience as our brain tries to protect us from harm.

Often, chronic pain is the result of multiple events rather than a single injury or disease. A history of trauma—physical or emotional—is more common among people who develop chronic pain than in the wider population, which means that feelings of depression and anxiety are often more prevalent.

> **Persistent pain actually rewires our brain.**

Pain interferes with sleep for most people, and conversely, poor sleep compounds their pain and related fatigue. Furthermore, the combination of chronic pain and poor sleep impacts both memory and concentration. Daily activities—at work, at home, and at leisure—are strongly affected by this perfect storm. Stressful situations become more difficult to handle, and relationships can become distant or strained.

The net result is profound suffering that often includes reduced mobility, loss of strength, immune impairment with increased susceptibility to disease, dependence on medication, and less ability to participate in enjoyable and meaningful activities with loved ones and our communities. In short, chronic pain can wreak havoc on life—leading to feelings of helplessness and hopelessness. But it doesn't have to be this way. To find relief and reclaim a vital life, it's important to recognize the emerging scientific understanding about the complex nature of chronic pain.

No Brain, No Pain

At some point you've probably felt that your pain was dismissed—and that you were belittled—when someone said, "Your pain is all in your head." While that statement is true, it doesn't mean you're crazy or that your pain isn't real. However, it's the *neurology*, not the *psychology*, of pain that's "all in your head." If you had no brain, you'd have no pain.

Most people have a rather fuzzy and outdated understanding of how pain occurs and of what is really going on in the mind and body of someone in chronic pain. Unfortunately, even many health care providers have not kept up to date with the rapid scientific advances that have shed new light on the complex neurobiology of pain during the last twenty-five years.

> **Pain is all in your head…neurologically.**

Yet despite its complexity, the essence of pain is quite simple and straightforward: *Pain functions as an alarm system.* Pain occurs whenever the brain determines that danger exists and that action is needed to reduce the perceived danger (Butler and Moseley

2013). If your hand accidentally touches a hot skillet, for example, instantaneously you'll feel burning sensations that prompt you to move your hand away from the skillet. If you step on a piece of glass, sharp sensations quickly alert you that you've been cut and need to be careful where you step next.

Both of these examples involve tissue damage: a burn on your hand in the first case, a cut on your foot in the second. However, pain can also be triggered by events that do *not* involve actual physical damage to your body. In fact, *whenever the pain alarm system prompts your brain to perceive a threat, you will feel hurt, regardless of how real that threat is*. The most striking example of how pain can be entirely separate from actual damage to your body is the common phenomenon of phantom pain, whereby people who lose a limb or other body part report excruciating pain in the region that is no longer there.

In contrast, it's also possible to *not* feel any pain, even if you've been badly hurt. If your brain calculates that an injury—even a severe one—is not the most important threat you face, then you may experience little or no pain. For example, soldiers injured on the battlefield often don't feel pain until a day or two later, after they've escaped or been rescued. And it's not uncommon for athletes who have suffered major injuries during a competition to not feel any pain until after the game has ended.

Typical Temporary Pain

The major insight to glean from these examples is this: "*It is the brain that decides whether something hurts or not, 100% of the time, with NO exceptions*" (Butler and Moseley 2013, 17). But how does the brain reach its conclusions? This is where the complexity begins. In the following pages we'll provide a summary of the mechanics. (For a more thorough explanation, please see the online chapter "More About Pain," available as part of the free digital resources that complement this book, along with guided audio meditations and video instruction, at http://www.newharbinger.com/43287.)

The pain process begins at the cellular level in millions of nerve cells called *nociceptors* (literally, "harm receptors") that are distributed throughout our body. When any of these neurons detects something that could cause harm, it transmits electrical impulses that signal "potential danger" into our spinal cord, which carries messages to and from our brain. If the incoming danger signals are strong enough, they open a biochemical "pain gate," which passes the signals up into the brain, and we begin to experience pain. But if the signals are weaker, this pain gate doesn't open and we won't feel pain.

Here's an example of how this works. Imagine you're on vacation in a city you've always wanted to visit. You embark on a long walking tour wearing a brand-new pair of shoes.

During the first hour of your walk, you notice some stiffness in your shoes, but you're having a great time and ignore the slight sensations. All the while, however, pressure-sensitive neurons in your feet are sending "danger" signals to your spinal cord that release a special chemical into the gap (or synapse) between two neurons. As you continue to walk, these chemicals will reach a level that opens the biochemical pain gate and delivers a danger message to your brain.

At this point, you will start to feel some pain, usually mild. Your conscious experience of this pain will include two main parts: a sensory one that relays the location and intensity of the danger sensations in your feet, and an emotional one, conveying the extent to which these sensations are interpreted as "bad" or unpleasant. If the sensations are sufficiently intense and unpleasant, then you will likely decide to either end your walk early or change into more comfortable shoes. If they are not so intense or unpleasant, you may decide you can tolerate the discomfort till the end of the tour.

While this example illustrates the typical temporary pain process, there are many ways this experience can be altered. One example involves specialized brain chemicals that can descend from the brain and block danger signals. This is part of the brain's "danger management" system, which involves the release of so-called "happy hormones"—such as *endorphins* (the body's own opioids) and *serotonin*—to counteract the danger signals in the spinal cord (Butler and Moseley 2013). This might occur if your walk includes a visit to a museum displaying your favorite painting. Your delight at seeing this masterpiece may trigger the release of happy hormones, which closes the biochemical pain gate so that your pain "disappears." Gazing at the beautiful painting, you might feel no pain in your feet.

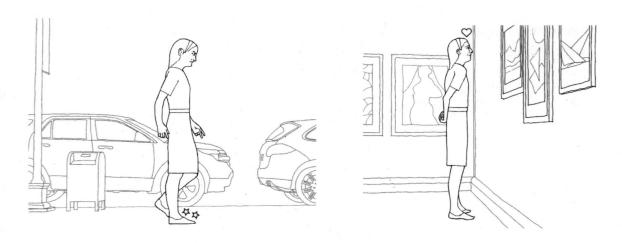

Pain signals can be dampened by the experience of something you enjoy.

And even if the danger signals do reach your brain, additional agents can alter how these signals are handled. As your brain attempts to interpret the signal's meaning, it must take into account millions of other simultaneously arriving signals and also compare them to its memory bank of past signal patterns. This activates what neuroscientists call the *pain neuromatrix*—a complex network spread across dozens of brain areas that are electrically and chemically linked together (Melzack 1999). Similar to a military situation involving signs of impending attack, as neural alarms go off warning "Danger! Incoming!," the pain neuromatrix team assesses where the threat is coming from and what the potential damage could be, and also compares the situation with memories of similar scenarios and evaluates readiness to respond.

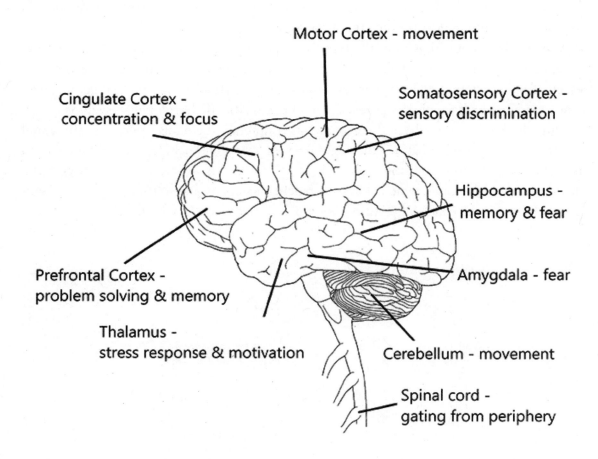

Motor Cortex - movement

Cingulate Cortex - concentration & focus

Somatosensory Cortex - sensory discrimination

Hippocampus - memory & fear

Prefrontal Cortex - problem solving & memory

Amygdala - fear

Thalamus - stress response & motivation

Cerebellum - movement

Spinal cord - gating from periphery

Brain areas involved in the "pain neuromatrix."

To assess the threat, our brain relies on various thought processes—including our beliefs and memories—to either boost or curtail transmission of incoming danger signals. For example, a belief that "It will be okay after a while" would decrease the rate of incoming danger signals. In contrast, memories of past painful experiences could directly activate new pain sensations—which could increase your pain, even in the absence of any new danger signals (Bayer et al. 1998).

Your outlook can also affect your pain—so if you expect something to hurt, it likely will, or vice versa. For example, if you anticipate that climbing a flight of stairs will "kill" your knees, just approaching a staircase may increase your pain. However, if you must walk up a flight of stairs to enter your beloved son's apartment, you may be so excited at the prospect of an enjoyable visit that your knees could feel fine despite the climb.

These examples illustrate how *our thoughts, emotions, expectations, and beliefs can have a profound impact on our perception of pain.* This won't come as a complete surprise if you've ever felt relief from a headache by watching an entertaining movie, or if you've coped with a toothache during a dental procedure by listening to your favorite music.

Take a few moments right now to recall a time when pain you were experiencing temporarily intensified because of where you were, who you were with, or what you were doing. Next, consider an example of when your pain temporarily got better because of where you were, who you were with, or what you were doing. Write down below examples of both experiences.

_____

_____

_____

_____

_____

Last, it's important to realize that when our brain determines we're in danger, it activates more than just the pain neuromatrix. The brain's "danger alert" also activates additional bodily systems that are part of the fight-or-flight response, which is designed to help us do battle or run away from harm. This means that our breathing and heart rate speed up, our muscles tense, and our blood pressure rises as our body revs up to deal with danger.

When the danger is over, our nervous system is designed to calm down our physiology. Unfortunately, in our tense, modern world, it's common for many people to remain in fight-or-flight mode, which means that our systems don't relax and instead remain activated over long periods of time. This kind of "hyperarousal" can lead to a cascade of stress-related disorders, including hypertension, type 2 diabetes, and heart attacks. Chronic hyperarousal is also a primary culprit in the onset of chronic pain.

How Temporary Pain Becomes Chronic

As pain persists for several months and becomes chronic, it gradually develops into a complex, *largely self-sustaining* network centered in the brain. Such pain is distinct from the original injury or condition that provoked the pain, and it often develops *despite the healing of damaged tissues.* This means that even after your body has healed, you may still feel pain—not because there is any damage but because your brain has become "wired" for pain.

Indeed, leading scientific experts propose that *chronic pain should be understood and treated as a distinct disease that is quite different from temporary pain caused by tissue damage* (Apkarian, Hashmi, and Baliki 2011). Brain scans of people suffering from chronic pain show that their brain "lights up" in different areas than are activated in people who are experiencing temporary pain (Wood 2010).

> **Once pain has become chronic, your brain is actually suffering from faulty wiring.**

Once pain has become chronic, your brain tries to protect you from injury but is actually suffering from faulty wiring. In other words, the brain has made a big mistake—it's now functioning like a car alarm system that has become so sensitive that even small movements from a breeze trigger a loud, endlessly repeating alarm (Butler and Moseley 2013).

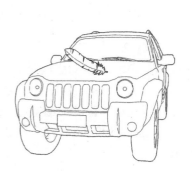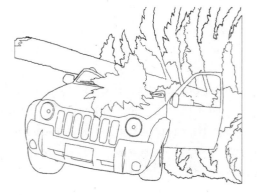

Chronic pain is like a car alarm gone haywire.

What Is Yoga—And How Can It Relieve Pain?

Yoga is an ancient discipline that has been practiced in India and other Asian countries for thousands of years. The word *yoga* comes from one of humanity's oldest languages, Sanskrit, and literally means to "yoke" or "unite." The practice is designed to unite many things. At the most basic level, yoga helps unite our body and mind. In actuality, our mind and body are never separate. But many of us are often *unaware* of the fundamental connections between what we think, feel, and do on the one hand, and how our bodies function on the other.

We also often lose touch with how our individual lives are linked to the greater world around us and with the deep-down goodness and wholeness that we all carry within ourselves. Yoga opens us to a conscious experience of these connections and—guided by that clear insight—the experience of greater happiness and less suffering.

For several decades, research into yoga's positive effects on chronic pain and other ailments has been growing exponentially. In addition to our studies, many other scientists have confirmed the benefits of yoga on persistent pain, including among individuals with osteoarthritis, migraines, carpal tunnel syndrome, kidney failure, and back pain (Garfinkel et al. 1994, 1998; John et al. 2007; Williams et al. 2009; Yurtkuran et al. 2007).

Notably, our work was the first to demonstrate that people with chronic pain can "rewire" the faulty circuitry in their brain by using the tools of yoga to restore a healthier pain response (Carson et al. 2016).

Research has also identified specific health benefits of yoga that contribute to improvements in chronic pain and related symptoms, including:

- an increased ability to *relax* deeply,

- a feeling of enhanced physical and mental *invigoration,* and

- a greater capacity to *accept* and adapt to our life challenges.

Relaxation

The *relaxation response* is the physiologic opposite of the fight-or-flight stress response. When stress is triggered, hormones are released that cause our breathing to become more rapid and shallow, heart rate and blood pressure to increase, muscles to tighten, and other changes that can amplify pain.

In contrast, during the relaxation response that yoga induces, our breath slows and deepens, heart rate lowers, blood pressure decreases, muscle tension eases, and other positive changes occur as the body shifts into a calm, healing mode. Studies show that the systematic deep bodily relaxation that yoga produces is associated not only with relief of pain but with reduction in other stress-related symptoms such as fatigue, poor sleep, emotional distress, and hot flashes (Telles et al. 2013; Telles, Reddy, and Nagendra 2000; Villemure and Bushnell 2002).

Invigoration

While it might seem paradoxical, yoga can be both relaxing and invigorating at the same time. Research confirms what yoga practitioners have always known: yoga has an invigorating effect on mental clarity and physical energy (Wood 1993). Feeling more invigorated makes it easier and less tiring to do everyday tasks, and that is typically accompanied by greater engagement in enjoyable and valued activities. The net effect of invigoration on pain is that we hurt less, are less limited by pain, and are less preoccupied with it.

Acceptance

When confronted with something unpleasant—whether a minor parking ticket or a major health challenge such as chronic pain—our mind commonly spins with resistance: "This is unfair! This can't be happening to me!" Yet all the effort we put into resistance typically increases our suffering.

A healthy sense of acceptance—to "let it be" for the time being—can help us break out of these negative autopilot reactions. Acceptance means "being willing to have the experience you are already having, versus resisting and struggling to escape from your own experience" (Hayes, Strosahl, and Wilson 1999). But accepting the reality of what is happening does not mean throwing our hands in the air and giving up. Instead, when we avoid wasting energy on resistance, we can see the truth of our circumstances more clearly and focus on constructive ways to deal with the situation. Research into the benefits of acceptance confirms its positive effects on chronic pain, anxiety, and depression—and that acceptance leads to fewer health care visits and prescription medications (McCracken et al. 2004; Hayes et al. 2006).

> **Suffering = Pain x Resistance**

Yoga Is Not Just a Workout

Over the past several decades, as yoga postures have become popularized in Western countries, the term "yoga" is typically used to refer to the physical aspect of the much fuller discipline. And it's certainly true that yoga postures—when appropriately tailored to specific conditions—can be helpful for improving pain.

However, posture practice is just one of yoga's many beneficial tools, so equating "yoga" with "posture" is not only inaccurate, it neglects the richness of the many other practices rooted in this ancient tradition. In fact, the Sanskrit word for posture is *asana,* which literally means "seat." This is because *traditionally, yoga has primarily been a discipline of seated meditation.* Yoga postures were originally cultivated to help practitioners become healthy and strong enough to remain comfortable during long periods of seated meditation.

Mindful Yoga, in keeping with the ancient tradition, centers on five main types of practices, each of which includes a variety of specific skills. These practices are briefly described below, then covered more thoroughly in subsequent chapters.

Postures

The practice of doing yoga poses (*asana*) has an overall toning effect on the body and can build strength, enhance flexibility, release tension, and improve balance and physical function—all of which can contribute to pain relief. In doing yoga postures, it is key to keep in mind the classical recommendation that "posture should embody steadiness and ease" (Hartranft 2003)." Mindful Yoga uses gentle postures and encourages a compassionate, curious approach—taking each movement to a point of challenge but not strain. But perhaps the most unique and potentially beneficial aspect of Mindful Yoga is the manner in which mindfulness is applied to the practice of yoga postures.

The term "mindfulness" has become increasingly popular in recent years and is sometimes misunderstood to mean "careful" or "considerate" or even "slow." However mindfulness actually refers to the open and non-judgmental, moment-to-moment awareness that is a fundamental capacity we all have (Kabat-Zinn 1990). Mindfulness can be practiced anytime, anywhere—even when we are feeling scattered, or moving quickly, or not thinking about much at all.

Learning to move mindfully—with a sense of kind curiosity, and without judgment—can be transformative for people used to our Western culture's "striving and pushing" mindset. Mindful Yoga also helps people recognize that the "undoing"—learning to recognize and release physical and mental tension—is as important as the doing. And learning to move in ways that challenge—without strain—in yoga postures can profoundly affect how you move through your daily activities.

Regardless of whether you are moving gently or more vigorously, yoga postures offer myriad opportunities for developing awareness that supports a healthier relationship to your body. Take a moment right now and notice how your body is positioned. Might there be a way you could sit or recline that might bring more ease? Richer dimensions of this practice open up as you learn to pay attention to both skillful bodily movements and to the shifting sensations that accompany such movements. You may become aware of pleasurable currents of sensations as you move, or hold a certain posture, or during the final relaxation pose. Frequently, practitioners feel refreshed, invigorated, and more at ease at the end of practice, which can be enjoyed well beyond the practice session.

> **Mindful Yoga helps refine our relationship to sensation through awareness.**

Likewise, integrating mindful awareness and related yogic principles into posture practice transforms the activity of "doing poses" into a forum for becoming aware of, and freeing yourself from, subtle patterns of reactivity to pain and other sensations. For example, if you notice that stress reactions—such as shallow breathing, excessive muscle tension, and fearful or anxious thoughts—arise when you're trying to balance on one leg, you can learn to shift out of these habits by practicing different responses, such as slowing your breath, relaxing your face, or not buying into anxious thoughts.

As you refine your relationship to sensations moment by moment during your posture practice, and you focus attention on how sensations interact with your thoughts and emotional responses, you can gradually "rewire" your brain so that uncomfortable sensations are not interpreted as quite so threatening.

Meditation

The practice of meditation, called *dhyana*, works directly with how we use our attention and what we focus on. While there are many types of meditation, Mindful Yoga strongly emphasizes mindfulness meditation—an aspect that distinguishes it from most yoga styles available today. During mindfulness meditation, you learn to better attune your attention to a variety of present-moment experiences, step by step, including noticing the natural movement of your breath, noticing sounds as they arise, noticing sensations as they appear, and noticing thoughts as they stream by—all while you remain aware of *simple being,* or noticing your own sense of presence right here, right now.

Substantial research supports the pain-relieving effects of mindfulness meditation, which calms the nervous system, strengthens focusing abilities, and clarifies mental processes (Grant 2014). Meditation can also be very helpful for how you handle daily tasks and challenges. Importantly, mindfulness meditation offers insights into your habitual patterns of thoughts, feelings, bodily reactions, and interactions with others, which can help you better recognize choices that contribute to your well-being versus choices that increase pain and suffering.

For example, once you have gained an understanding of how pain is produced by your nervous system, you can learn to work more skillfully with how you think about pain, how you handle emotional reactions to your discomfort, how you breathe, and how you engage in various activities. As you make more skillful choices, this will contribute to a greater sense of safety in your nervous system and tamp down the danger signals that ramp up the pain in your brain. As a result, you will begin to feel better and suffer less.

Breathing

Breath regulation, called *pranayama*, involves techniques for attending to and guiding your breath. How we breathe has a powerful effect on both mind and body—which won't come as a surprise to women who have used breathing techniques to manage pain during childbirth. Specific breathing practices, including simply resting into the natural breath, can help with pain, stress, anxiety, and other distressing symptoms (Busch et al. 2012; Dhruva et al. 2012).

Self-Study

Mindful Yoga stands out from many contemporary yoga styles in its emphasis on yogic philosophical foundations, such as simple being (*sat*), mindful awareness (*chit*), and love (*ananda*). A key yogic principle is self-study (*svadhyaya*), which involves studying wisdom teachings and applying them to your own direct experience of life. As you practice this type of self-inquiry, it sheds further light on your habits of body and mind, which is the first step in making changes that can move you in the direction of wholeness, better health, and less pain.

"Keeping the Company of Truth"

Part of our Mindful Yoga program focuses on *satsanga*, which means "communing with the truth." This practice includes being truthful with yourself and others about what you are experiencing, and learning from your yoga practice and your life. More specific, this will involve journaling—writing down your thoughts and feelings in this workbook. To benefit from this practice, it's essential to "keep the company of truth"—writing to learn from your experiences rather than to impress anyone. Journaling is one of the oldest forms of self-inquiry and self-expression. It has many benefits, including helping you see more clearly what impacts your pain and how to apply that insight into your daily life.

Inner Transformation

As you engage in these Mindful Yoga practices over time, you will discover that your awareness of yourself and of life's possibilities will grow broader, deeper, and clearer. A fundamental shift will gradually develop in how you relate to your "self." You will begin to recognize that "whatever you think, say or do, a sense of immutable and affectionate being remains as the ever-present background of the mind" (Nisargadatta 1985). You can discover an internal refuge that is deeply nourishing and, importantly, always available to you. This inner refuge is especially helpful when dealing with difficult challenges such as chronic pain. As your insight grows, you will likely find yourself more at peace and more able to access the equanimity, courage, and patience to "ride the waves" of life, however tumultuous.

In summary, the benefits that Debbie discovered through Mindful Yoga are not rare. We have worked with hundreds of people who credit Mindful Yoga with decreasing their pain and reducing or eliminating their need for opioid medications. Mindful Yoga has also improved their mood and mental outlook, giving them better sleep, extra energy, and boosts in their strength, balance, and flexibility. A complete yoga program that integrates posture, meditation, and breathing practices with the study of yogic wisdom can reunite you with an unfathomable source of energy—and bring about a truly liberating shift in how you relate to pain and to life itself.

How to Use This Book

In *Relax into Yoga for Chronic Pain*, we present an eight-week program designed to give you the information and tools you need to feel better, move better, sleep better, function better, and reduce or eliminate your need for pain medication. Based on the series of classes used in Jim and Kimberly's scientific studies, this workbook is a step-by-step guide to skillfully using yoga techniques to manage pain.

Each chapter, or Week, focuses on a specific concern—such as stress, pain, difficult emotions, and fatigue—and presents a set of skills to help deal with these issues. Each Week also includes instruction in specific practices of gentle movement, breathing, and meditation, which are illustrated and supported with downloadable audio recordings and streaming videos available at http://www.newharbinger.com/43287.

We recommend that you focus on one chapter each week, giving yourself time to read and assimilate the material, plus experience the practices. At the start of Weeks 2 through 8 is a brief reflection section that invites you to review what you have learned before proceeding and addresses common questions and concerns that may arise.

Each Week builds on the yoga foundations and practices presented in previous Weeks. To continue your progress, it's vital that you develop the skills, week by week, that will progressively propel you toward the harbor of greater resiliency and pain relief. Simply reading this book without doing the practices is not likely to be noticeably helpful for your pain or overall quality of life.

Given that daily practice is vital to achieve optimal results, we recommend that you schedule a daily practice session into your life. As you begin, fifteen to twenty minutes a day will be enough to notice a difference. Avoid rushing. With patience, persistence, and regular practice, Mindful Yoga can be a transformative experience.

WEEK·1

Riding the Waves: Beginning Your Mindful Yoga Journey

You must live in the present, launch yourself on every wave.

—Henry David Thoreau

It's a common misconception that yoga primarily means doing postures—often involving complex twisting, balancing, and going upside down. This can be daunting for many of us, especially if we live with chronic pain and find everyday activities like getting dressed or climbing stairs quite challenging. So please, rest assured, that you don't need to be able to sit cross-legged on the floor, touch your toes, or even get out of bed to practice yoga and reap its many benefits. All you need to practice yoga is breath and attention.

In fact, cultivating moment-to-moment attention, and noticing the effects of breath, are key elements of our Mindful Yoga approach, which centers on a process we call *riding the waves.* Just as a skilled ferryman learns to pay attention to the current, wind, and weather to expertly ride the restless ocean waves, Mindful Yoga invites us to pay attention to the sensations in our bodies, the emotions in our hearts, and the thoughts in our minds—so we can skillfully ride the sometimes tumultuous waves of our lives.

At the heart of Mindful Yoga is the recognition that, while many things around us constantly change, at the core of each of us there is an unchanging subtle presence and goodness. Enhancing our awareness of both—what changes and what remains the same—can help us better navigate the waves of pain, fatigue, and difficult emotions that can threaten to sink us.

For example, you've probably noticed that—in any musical performance—the first musical notes emerge out of a moment of initial

> **All you need to practice yoga is breath and attention.**

silence, and then, eventually, the final musical notes subside again into silence. The great composers intentionally and skillfully make use of the dynamic interplay between sounds and silence in their music.

Mindful Yoga is likewise focused on a dynamic interplay of two very distinct yet complementary processes: *Developing greater awareness of the ever-changing waves—the ups, downs, and shifts—that make up our life, along with enhanced awareness of the unchanging steadiness of our basic sense of being.* The tools of yoga—postures, meditation, breathing, and self-study—can help us learn to steady our boat and ride the waves of life so that we experience greater ease, joy, and pain relief.

Much more than a series of exercises, yoga is actually an approach to life that provides guidance on how to live skillfully and fruitfully. This is captured beautifully by our favorite traditional definition of yoga: Yoga is skill in action.

Ancient yogis recognized an important truth that modern scientific evidence supports:

> **Yoga is skill in action.**

Our thoughts and feelings often have a profound influence on our health and well-being. Yoga centers on cultivating awareness of what's going on in our bodies, minds, and emotional hearts. It offers a variety of skills to help us navigate the inevitable ups and downs of life, including the complex challenge of chronic pain.

Mindful awareness—that is, moment-to-moment nonjudgmental recognition of what's happening in the present moment—is the key to skillful living, and all elements of our Mindful Yoga program are designed to help you become more aware, connected, and at ease in your daily life.

Not surprising, in our busy, stressful world, many of us become so wrapped up in worrying about what we need to get done—for our jobs, families, and communities—that we often become disconnected from what's going on right under our noses. We may let our mind agonize about the past or worry about the future, become disconnected from our feelings, and sometimes even ignore signals from our body that indicate it needs support.

For example, you may disregard a "twinge" in your knee until one morning you are unable to walk, or you may suppress feelings of sadness because you've been told that "it's time to get over the loss" of a loved one. Even the common experience of driving somewhere and—when you've arrived at your destination—realizing that you can't remember any of the drive, illustrates the "mindlessness" or *distracted attention* that is so common in our fast-paced world.

In contrast, yoga invites us to notice moment by moment what's going on physically, emotionally, and mentally—with a sense of kindness and compassion—so that we can reconnect with our inner resources and more skillfully manage any challenges we encounter.

As a result, rather than mindlessly battling the ever-changing waves of life, yoga teaches us how to steer skillfully.

Foundations of Yoga Practice

Mindful Yoga is grounded in five principles that are recognizable as universal values of a life well lived:

- Mindful awareness

- Simple being

- Acceptance

- Love

- Riding the waves

None is independent of the others—they are all interrelated, like facets of a five-sided diamond.

Mindful Awareness

Awareness (*chit*) is our innate capacity to directly encounter and observe our own experience. *Mindful awareness* is the practice of watching yourself in your daily life with alert interest—purposely noticing your thoughts, feelings, sensations, and actions—with the intention to understand rather than to judge (Nisargadatta 1985). This process provides the raw material for learning to live skillfully.

Right now your attention is focused on reading these words, and your experience is being shaped by your mind reflecting on the meaning of what you are reading. However, if you were to put down this book and move to look out a window, your visual field would be different, and your thoughts and emotions would likely to be different too. Our awareness reflects what we focus on—whether our inner or outer experiences, or both.

Awareness is always in the background of our life. We may be aware that we are stressed, or aware that we are at ease, or aware that we are having a hard time focusing. What we may *not* be as aware of is *how we are using our attention* and *the way our attention shapes our experience of everything in life, including pain.*

For example, if we focus constantly on what we are afraid may happen, such as our pain getting worse, we are haunted by a sense of fear. If we are constantly focusing our attention on what we want but don't have, our experience is dominated by a sense of lack. If, on the other hand, we focus primarily on the people and the situations we love and enjoy, our daily experience is suffused with love and joy.

Since we are always paying attention to some aspects of our experience while ignoring others, Mindful Yoga places strong emphasis on *what we attend* to, as well as the *quality of our attention,* in daily life. As we refine our attentional abilities—noticing thoughts, feelings, sensations, and actions—we begin to learn firsthand what choices contribute to our well-being, and which ones lead to more pain, conflict, and suffering.

Simple Being

"Simple being" (*sat*) refers to your familiar, immediate sense of being present—your awareness that "I am" (Maharshi 2000; Nisargadatta 1985). You may not have realized it before, but the sense "I am" is always present at any given moment, across all your life experiences. Throughout your lifespan—regardless of age-related bodily changes (childhood, adolescence, adulthood), or varied emotional changes (happy, sad, angry), or changes in your thoughts (remembering, anticipating, commenting)—*this basic aspect of you has never changed.* As you cultivate awareness of simple being, you will begin to discover that connecting to this unchanging part of yourself provides a powerful doorway to deep inner resources—of wholeness, ease, energy, love, and insight.

Simple Being: Just Present

Right now, with clear but relaxed attention, begin to take notice of your sense of just being present, right here, in the midst of whatever else you may be experiencing—whatever you're seeing or hearing around you, or sensing in your body. This simple sense of presence, of "I am," is like a mirror: All kinds of activities can be simultaneously reflected in a mirror, but the mirror itself doesn't change.

Once you've identified simple being, it's valuable to take greater notice of this "steady anchor point" in the midst of your daily life. You'll find that this simple, stable, unchanging part of you is very reliable: it's a vantage point you can come back to, to get centered and find your bearings in all kinds of situations.

Acceptance

Life can be difficult, and experiences such as illness, loss, and the death of loved ones can't be avoided. Internal unpleasant experiences—including worrisome thoughts, distressing emotions, and uncomfortable sensations—also cannot be completely avoided. "Acceptance" (*tapas*) in this context is your willingness to "let it be" and have the experience you are already having—to face and learn from whatever adversities you encounter—instead of denying or struggling to escape from your own experiences (Hayes, Follett, and Linehan 2004).

Accepting a difficult situation doesn't mean giving up—rather, it means avoiding unnecessary struggle and not wasting energy on wishing that things were different from how they actually are. By cultivating acceptance—through the practice of neither grasping after nor pushing away experiences—we struggle less. We then find greater calm and are better able to access the courage, flexibility, and patience to face adversities. However, acceptance can't be forced or artificial: "I accept, because I *should*" doesn't work. And acceptance is not a one-time decision but rather a moment-by-moment, day-by-day process, like continually tending to a garden.

The familiar serenity creed outlines the essence of acceptance: "May I be granted the serenity to *accept* the things I cannot change; courage to change the things I can; and wisdom to know the difference." Acceptance requires discernment—recognizing the difference between what we can change and what we cannot.

As you read this, you may want to ask yourself: Is there something I am struggling to make happen in my life, something that's really not working and only making me suffer more?

For example, if you have not been employed for a while due in part to chronic pain, you may be thinking a lot about going back to work, even though that seems very difficult to achieve and sustain. So is there some other goal you can channel your energies toward that is likely to be more achievable and rewarding?

Even more important is moment-to-moment acceptance. For example, if an accident on the highway has stalled traffic and there is no alternative route available, rather than complaining and fueling emotional reactions to the situation, we can practice accepting the circumstances of the moment.

Love

Within each of us is a deep-down goodness, a fundamental capacity for love (*ananda*), although this capacity may not always be apparent. Love encompasses both an inner feeling and the expression of that feeling in actions. While hard to define, love takes many forms that are easily recognized, such as expressions of caring, kindness, receptivity, and sensitivity in our actions. As in most wisdom traditions, yoga emphasizes that love begins with loving yourself.

Love has probably been best described by sages from various wisdom traditions. Here is a brief collection of wise sayings about love. We suggest that after reading them, you pick one that speaks clearly to you. Then spend a couple of minutes rereading this quote, while doing your best to tune in to any feelings of love that arise as you contemplate its meaning.

"Being deeply loved by someone gives you strength, while loving someone deeply gives you courage." —Lao Tzu, Chinese philosopher

"Love your neighbor as yourself." —(Leviticus 19:18, Hebrew Torah)

"Let the beauty we love be what we do. There are hundreds of ways to kneel and kiss the ground." —Rumi, Persian poet

"A new commandment I give to you, that you love one another, as I have loved you." —Jesus Christ (John 13:34)

"Radiate boundless love towards the entire world—above, below, and across—unhindered, without ill will." —Gautama the Buddha (Metta Sutta)

"Love your life. Perfect your life. Beautify all things in your life." —Tecumseh, Shawnee chief

Riding the Waves

"Riding the waves" is a traditional yogic metaphor that may sound unrelated to healing chronic pain (Faulds 2005). However, what we know from the most advanced fields of science, including quantum physics, is that everything in the universe actually does vibrate in wavelike patterns—sound waves, light waves, ocean waves, seismic waves, brain waves, even gravity waves. Many of these waves are difficult to perceive.

If you've ever blown into a dog whistle and watched your dog respond to a sound that you don't hear, you know it's because canine ears hear sound wave frequencies that humans can't detect. Similarly, what appears to your eyes as pitch-black darkness is not so to cats, whose eyes discern light wave frequencies that we can't see. And solidly appearing objects around you—such as the furniture in the room you're in right now—if examined with a powerful electron microscope, are revealed as composed of subatomic "wavicles" vibrating at various frequencies (Valdivia 2014).

With practice, we can attune attention to wave patterns that are central to our experience of life. All sensations—including pain and pleasure, and all emotions and thoughts—are constantly moving in wavelike rhythms, arising, cresting, and eventually subsiding. The definition of yoga as "skill in action" (*karmasu kaushalam*) means learning to skillfully navigate, or ride, the many types of waves that we encounter in life.

While sometimes we may wish that particular waves, such as pain flares, would stop, the truth is that we can't really stop the waves of life. However, we can learn to more skillfully ride these waves, and we may also be able to stop fueling certain waves. As a result, we experience greater calm, freedom, and joy. The overall aim of yoga practice is to help us learn to navigate all the varied waves of life, be they big and rough, or gentle and quiet.

Riding the Waves = Living Skillfully

Life is a dynamic, ever-changing experience. Some changes we find pleasant and desirable, while others may be adverse and difficult. By attuning your attention to the wavelike patterns—appearing, peaking, fading—of everything you encounter, you can find your balance and keep your poise amid the tumult of life's ever-changing waves.

We invite you, right now, to experiment with riding one of the simplest, yet most vital, waves of life.

Begin with your eyes opened or closed. First, attune your attention carefully to the rhythm of your breath. Let your breath move at its natural pace, without trying to control it.

Can you feel the inhalation phase? Do you notice a brief pause, accompanied by a sensation of completion, at the top of the inhalation? Can you feel the exhalation happening? Is there another brief pause at the end of the exhalation, before the next inhalation begins?

Stay attuned in this way for at least five breaths. Then notice how you feel. You might feel extra alert and quite aware that you are alive. Welcome to riding the waves of breath—and riding the waves of life.

Foundations of Yoga Practice

Mindful Awareness: watching yourself in your daily life with alert interest—noticing bodily sensations, thoughts, feelings, and actions—with the intention to understand rather than to judge

Simple Being: your immediate sense of "I am," of existing and being present, at any given moment; a reliable point you can come back to, to get centered and find your bearings

Acceptance: being willing to face whatever adversities you must encounter, versus resisting and struggling to escape your own experience

Love: the deep-down goodness within all of us that is the basis for qualities such as kindness and caring

Riding the Waves: living skillfully; finding your balance and keeping your poise amid the tumult of life's ever-changing waves

Andrea's Story

As a high school PE teacher, Andrea had been active all her life. Yet just after menopause, she was diagnosed with osteoporosis and placed on a medication that unfortunately had serious side effects. By the time she was nearing retirement, this tall, slender woman's bones had become so brittle that her left femur snapped. She underwent surgery to place a steel rod in her thigh. Once she had fully recovered, she was able to walk normally again. However, she experienced persistent pain along the length of her leg that became more intense as each day went on.

Andrea enrolled in our Mindful Yoga course at the suggestion of her physical therapist. She was apprehensive about being able to do even gentle yoga postures, but she was pleasantly surprised at how accessible the practice was during the first class. The following week, along with doing the recommended posture and breath exercises at home, Andrea also did the informal practice of pausing a few times each day to observe her breath for a short while. She soon discovered that she had a habit of holding her breath and keeping her breath short and shallow. Moreover, she realized that during those moments her pain tended to be worse and was accompanied by stronger tension along her left hip and leg.

As a PE teacher, Andrea knew that this pattern of restricted breathing and physical tension was a reaction to feeling stressed. So she started doing additional mini breathing practices

throughout her day, and she found that afterward not only was her breathing more full and relaxed, but her tension and pain eased too. As she shared this experience during the second class, she said, "For the last couple of days my pain has been the best it's been in months!"

Mindful Yoga Practices

Breath Practice

How we breathe has a powerful effect on both mind and body. When we become stressed or frightened, we often unconsciously tighten our abdomen and use secondary breathing muscles of the chest, neck, and upper back, resulting in a fast, shallow breathing pattern.

When we relax, the abdomen softens and we are able to more efficiently allow the diaphragm muscle to facilitate a fuller, slower, and more rhythmical breath. Located beneath the lowest two ribs and spanning the width of the torso, the diaphragm is the primary muscle for respiration, responsible for 75 percent of all respiratory effort. When our breathing is mainly diaphragmatic, our lungs are able to expand more completely. This means that more oxygen is taken in with each breath. In addition, the fuller upward movement of the diaphragm on exhalation allows the lungs to empty more completely of carbon dioxide.

The central breathing exercise we will teach you—Three-Part Breath—encourages the healthy mechanics of diaphragmatic breathing; it also counters the common habit of shallow or guarded breathing. Understanding how Three-Part Breath works and how to practice it will help you to calm your mind and also relax and revitalize your body.

Three-Part Breath focuses on three areas within the torso. The first is the lower level in the abdominal area under the navel. This is the area that we soften so that the diaphragm can descend and facilitate a full inhalation. The second area is the middle chest, or thoracic region around the ribs. Breathing into this area lifts your rib cage and allows the intercostal muscles between the ribs to expand. The third section is located around the area of the upper chest and just under the collar bones.

Good breathing creates more than just a transitory sense of well-being. It has major implications for our health. During Three-Part Breath, the rhythmical upward and downward movements of the diaphragm—combined with the outward and inward movements of the belly, rib cage, and upper chest—promote better blood flow, balance the autonomic nervous system, and pump the lymph more efficiently through the lymphatic system. This is critical, since the lymphatic system—which is an important part of the immune system—has no pump other than muscular movements, including the movements of breathing.

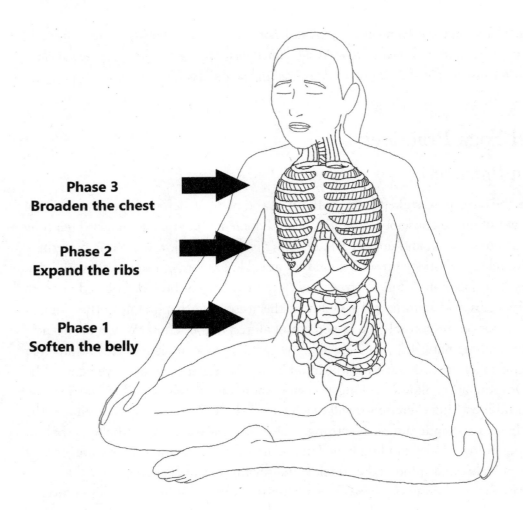

Phase 3
Broaden the chest

Phase 2
Expand the ribs

Phase 1
Soften the belly

Three-part Breath Practice

Studies indicate that diaphragmatic breathing creates a relaxed state by enhancing parasympathetic tone, which means this type of breathing supports the part of our nervous system that helps us recover from stress and threat. Breathing in this way has been demonstrated to have numerous therapeutic effects, including pain-relief (Martin et al. 2012) and improvements in sleep disturbance and anxiety in cancer patients receiving chemotherapy, of blood pressure in people with hypertension, and with hot flashes during menopause (Dhruva et al. 2012; Germaine and Freedman 1984).

Three-Part Breath

This breathing pattern can be done anywhere and anytime, multiple times a day or at night. While you can do this practice in any position—lying down, sitting in a chair, or standing—it's easiest to learn when you're lying down or sitting in a reclined position. Try this breath for a few moments (5 to 7 complete rounds) and then notice how you feel.

It's probably easiest to do this practice by following the Three-Part Breath guided audio at http://www.newharbinger.com/43287. Alternatively, you can guide yourself using the following instructions:

Part 1: Rest your hands on your belly, just below the navel. As you take your next breath in, let your belly soften and expand like a balloon. As you breathe out, let your belly sink. Repeat 3 times.

Part 2: Rest one hand on your ribs and one hand on your belly. With your next inhale, let your belly soften and allow your ribs to expand to the left and to the right. As you exhale, let everything sink. Repeat 3 times.

Part 3: Rest the hand that was on your ribs on your upper chest, just below your collarbones. As you breathe in, allow your belly to soften, your ribs to expand, and your upper chest to broaden. As you exhale, let everything relax back down. Spend a few moments in this three-part rhythm, letting the breath soften and nourish your body.

As this breath begins to feel more familiar, explore letting your breath be as full in your back body as in your front body. As you breathe into your belly, there is also a gentle expansion through your lower back; as the ribs of your front body expand, so do the ribs in your back body; and as your upper chest broadens, so does your upper back.

When you're ready to finish, just let your breath fall back into its natural rhythm. Notice the impact of Three-Part Breath.

Mindful Posture Sequences

Engaging in yoga poses that are safe and appropriate for your body can be very rewarding in a variety of ways. We've seen the posture practice help our students boost their strength and balance, enhance their fitness and flexibility, and improve their ability to do meaningful activities. Scientific studies have substantiated the many benefits of regularly practicing yoga poses (Buffart et al. 2012; Cramer, Lauche, and Langhorst 2013; Raub 2002; Villemure and Bushnell 2002; Wren et al. 2011; Yurtkuran et al. 2007).

Yet to fully appreciate the value of yoga poses, it's important to realize that this type of exercise is not simply about safe, healthy physical movement. Along with making our bodies stronger and more flexible, yoga poses, when done in a mindful manner, offer opportunities for *enhancing the strength and flexibility of our minds.*

Mindful Yoga invites us to develop a new awareness of—and relationship to—our bodily sensations, thought patterns, and emotional responses. Doing yoga poses in this manner allows us to become aware of—and free ourselves from—subtle patterns of reactivity and resistance, including anxious or irritated thoughts, shallow breathing, and widespread muscle tension, especially around areas that hurt.

Called "guarding," this common habit of unconsciously clenching muscles in an effort to protect vulnerable areas actually makes pain worse, as it increases sensitivity in the tissues as well as results in chronic stiffness, making fluid movement more difficult. At the end of yoga posture practice, it's common to feel refreshed and invigorated, with a sense of calm that often lingers. As we grow more familiar with these movements, our confidence in our ability to engage in other types of physical activities grows, and moving through our lives becomes more sustainable, meaningful, and enjoyable.

Formal and Informal Practices

To gain the most benefit from Mindful Yoga, it's helpful to do both formal and informal practices. The *formal practices*, which are done at specific times in specific ways, include the gentle posture sequences, the breath practices, and the meditations. These practices are invaluable for developing the skills that can bring more ease and pain relief.

Informal practices, on the other hand, are just as important but are spread throughout your day and woven into the fabric of daily life. For example, you might observe your breath when you are stopped at a traffic light, or bring your attention to thoughts that arise when your pain seems to worsen. This method of incorporating "micro-practices" helps to integrate the specific skills you are developing into your moment-to-moment experience of life. Journaling about these informal practices deepens your self-study so that you can more clearly see subtle aspects of your experience that you may otherwise overlook.

Week 1 Recommended Practice Schedule

Formal Practice

Record notes on the formal practice calendar. Jot down your practice times and observations on the weekly calendar provided at the end of this chapter.

Postures

Week 1 Yoga Posture Sequence. Turn to the "Mindful Yoga Posture Practices" section on page 133 and follow the instructions for Week 1; you can also follow along with the downloadable video available at http://www.newharbinger.com/43287. Practice every other day, at least three times this week. As you do the postures, simply notice waves of various bodily sensations: stretching, holding, releasing, tingling, and so on.

Breathing

Three-Part Breath. Practice each day (with or without the downloadable audio at http://www.newharbinger.com/43287).

Informal Practice

Self-study. Spend a few moments in the midst of daily life noticing your breath moving. Refrain from trying to change its spontaneous rhythm—discover what it's like to just notice the breath happening on its own.

Keeping the company of truth. On the following worksheet, describe what you observe and learn about your natural breathing pattern.

Keeping the Company of Truth: Riding the Waves of the Breath

Spend a few moments in the midst of daily life observing the arising, cresting, and subsiding of your breath, without attempting to alter its natural rhythm.	Did watching the waves of the breath seem to make any difference for you today? Describe what happened.
Day 1	
Day 2	
Day 3	
Day 4	
Day 5	
Day 6	
Day 7	

Week 1 Formal Practice—Beginning Your Mindful Yoga Journey

Record time spent in each practice. Note any observations.

	Breath Three-Part Breath	Postures Week 1	Observations What did you notice during or after practice?
Day 1 Time			
Notes			
Day 2 Time			
Notes			
Day 3 Time			
Notes			

	Breath Three-Part Breath	Postures Week 1	Observations What did you notice during or after practice?
Day 4 Time			
Notes			
Day 5 Time			
Notes			
Day 6 Time			
Notes			
Day 7 Time			
Notes			

Week 1 Review

Before proceeding further, let's review what you learned in Week 1.

First, practice Three-Part Breath for a few moments.

Next, turn to page 21 and review the "Foundations of Yoga Practice." Ask yourself, "Am I starting to understand why each of these foundations is potentially helpful and important?"

Next, turn to page 31 and review the "Week 1 Recommended Practice Schedule."

Were you able to do both the formal and informal practices as suggested?

_____

_____

What did you experience as a result of your practice—perhaps a sense of relaxation, calm, or well-being?

_____

_____

Did you notice any agitation or impatience?

_____

_____

Has your pain decreased or been more tolerable? Or has it remained unchanged?

_____

_____

Briefly describe how your yoga practices have affected you this week.

_____

_____

_____

_____

_____

Did any particular challenges arise that made practicing difficult? Common concerns at this stage are finding it hard to make time for practice and having expectations that didn't match your actual experience. If you didn't practice as much as you hoped, or you found practice difficult, know that you are in good company. Most people have similar challenges when they begin their yoga journey. Here are two common challenges and some suggestions for addressing them.

It's hard fitting practice into my life.

If you weren't able to do most of the recommended practices, what got in the way? If you tried to follow a regular schedule, remember that it's also important to be flexible and have a plan-B time to practice. On days when you can't do the full practice, just do what you can—even if it's just five to ten minutes. Even a short practice will bring some benefit and will help you establish a rhythm. Over time, most people begin to look forward to their practice because it brings a sense of relief and increased energy. When your daily practice becomes a welcome opportunity for self-care, making time becomes easier.

I'm feeling impatient and frustrated.

Learning anything new can be challenging. Moving in unfamiliar ways is no exception. When chronic pain has been part of your internal experience for a while, there will be some movements that feel really hard, disconnected, and sometimes even demoralizing. Be patient with yourself. Let go of any need to "master" the movements. Rather, allow yourself to become very curious about what you notice as you pay kind and careful attention to the experience, patiently retraining your nervous system one breath at a time.

WEEK 2

Riding the Waves of Attention

Do not undervalue attention: It means interest and also love.
To know, to do, to discover, or to create,
you must give your heart to it, which means attention.

—Nisargadatta Maharaj (Indian philosopher,
1897–1981)

How we use our attention—specifically what we choose to focus on—shapes our experience of everything in life, including pain. Jim often tells the following story to illustrate the importance of paying attention:

"Soon after Kimberly and I became engaged, I planned a special treat to celebrate her birthday. I knew she loved peaches, so I bought several beautiful Georgia peaches. Very excited, I cut up the juicy peaches while imagining how happy Kimberly would be with this surprise. When I placed that bowl of peaches topped with fresh whipped cream in front of her, Kimberly seemed delighted—until she brought the first spoonful to her lips and discovered the sharp edges of a peach pit shard in the spoon!

"Fortunately, she didn't break a tooth. But as you can imagine, I was shocked and embarrassed—and I have never forgotten that mistake. That day I learned in a very vivid way that *what counts most in any moment, no matter the situation, is how well we pay attention to what is actually happening.* I had the best of intentions as I was preparing those peaches, but instead of focusing on what my hands were actually doing, I was lost in my thoughts, anticipating how pleased Kimberly would be. However, no amount of good intentions can make up for lack of attention."

Here's another example of good intentions foiled through inattention. After a heavy snowfall, a middle-aged man with both chronic low-back pain and a good dose of stubbornness decided that, despite his recent lumbar surgery, he was going to shovel the driveway so his wife could get to work, just as he had always done. Several minutes into this demanding activity he began to feel a new twinge in his back, but he ignored it and kept on shoveling. By the time he had finished, his back was fully inflamed. He hardly slept that night, and it took him three full days of doing next to nothing before his pain backed off to a tolerable level. Again, his intentions had been good, but ignoring what needed careful attention literally backfired.

Attention Is Our Greatest Asset

Paying attention is an essential component of virtually everything we do. Consider driving a car. Almost all accidents—which often result in life-altering painful injuries, and even death—happen because of poor attention to the road. Lesser consequences include getting lost, missing an exit, and arriving late.

How about when you're responsible for looking after children? Kids often demand our attention, and if we don't pay attention, we can expect trouble—children can make poor decisions and end up hurting themselves or one another. Providing loving care for young ones means giving them your attention.

Another example is playing sports or games. When we are fully attentive, we tend to perform much better on a court or field and are much better at playing the right card or making the best move in a game. How do you feel about a teammate who is not paying attention and messes up in the middle of a good game?

We could go on and on about why attention is critical to our lives—when we're on the job, when we're with a loved one, when we're learning a new skill, and so on. In reality, *attention is our greatest asset*.

> **Attention can be likened to focusing a stage light into a spotlight that you use to highlight a particular portion of the stage.**

But what exactly do we mean by "attention"? The word comes from the Latin *tendere*, which means "to extend." What is it that we extend when we pay attention? We extend awareness—our ability to know and experience anything and everything that we encounter in life. So attention is the process of extending our awareness toward a certain object or activity.

Awareness itself can be compared to a powerful stage light that illumines everything that happens on a theater stage. Attention can be likened to focusing a stage light into a spotlight that you use to highlight a particular portion of the stage.

Challenges in Riding the Waves of Attention

Hopefully it's now clear that your ability to pay attention is critical to anything you want to do well. Yet, this most essential asset is often taken for granted, so that many of us often don't notice how we are using our attention. Instead, we slip into autopilot mode, and whatever habits of mind we have developed take over. Examples abound: Flaring your back when you lift a heavy object because you are busy thinking about something else instead of paying attention to good body mechanics; talking on your cellphone when getting into your car and then, halfway to your destination, realizing you left your walking cane at home. Unfortunately, when we are "missing in action" like this, we often unconsciously end up using our attention in ways that are unskillful or even harmful.

Neuroscientists describe several important characteristics of human attention. First, like everything in the universe, attention naturally fluctuates in a barely perceptible, wavelike pattern. In most people, this slight waxing and waning is not problematic, but larger attention variations are associated with attention-deficit disorders (Gilden and Hancock 2007). As anyone with attention-deficit issues will tell you, these difficulties are quite challenging. For all of us, attention problems are magnified by chronic pain. That's because pain signals tend to be perceived by our brains as more salient—that is, more important and urgently in need of our attention—than other stimuli. This contributes to significant attention problems, including difficulty in shifting one's focus, in most people experiencing persistent pain (Alshelh et al. 2018).

For example, if a person who is not experiencing pain goes to a movie and finds the only available seats are up a flight of stairs, the salience (importance) of climbing the stairs may be so minor that the person hardly notices. On the other hand, if you have chronic knee pain, just glancing up those stairs may totally capture your attention and even provoke such strong anticipatory pain that you may decide to skip the movie. If you repeatedly make that choice, and similar choices to avoid activities, then you will gradually but unknowingly condition your brain for activity avoidance through a process known as *neuroplasticity*.

Summed up as "neurons that fire together, wire together," neuroplasticity means that any two events that repeatedly occur together gradually become linked together neurologically, so that if one of these events happens, the other event is triggered in the brain (Doidge 2007). Over time, the urge to avoid activities in an effort to avoid pain will come to dominate your attention and thereby block your participation in many potentially enjoyable and valued activities.

Furthermore, in many people, via the same neuroplasticity conditioning, attention to pain sensations becomes neurologically linked with a sense of distress, accompanied by thoughts of wanting to escape the pain. Although this is a natural response, over time it sets up a negative feedback loop: Attention to pain triggers emotional distress and anxious thoughts, which further highlights the attentional spotlight on pain. This, in turn, magnifies your experience of pain, and, of course, feeling more pain fuels more distress and more thoughts about pain.

Apart from amplifying the pain itself, fixating attention on pain is problematic because mental flexibility is important for noticing, and thereby experiencing, sensations or emotions other than pain and distress. This means that even if you're doing something others find relaxing and soothing, such as getting a massage, you may not experience much relief because attention is so preoccupied with pain.

Attentional flexibility is also crucial for engaging in daily activities. You need to be able to turn attention to whatever it is you're doing. But if attention is so wrapped up in pain and distress that it can't be directed elsewhere for long, you are likely to feel constantly distracted from whatever you try to do—be it driving, conversing with someone, reading, watching TV, or anything else.

Given how important attention is to everything we experience in life, the primary purpose of all the Mindful Yoga practices—meditation, breathing, postures, and self-study— is to cultivate both stability and flexibility in how we use our attention. Learning to direct attention skillfully is the essence of mindful awareness and at the heart of coping better with chronic pain.

If you have started trying some of the Mindful Yoga practices, such as postures and Three-Part Breath, you may have begun to notice some changes already—such as feeling a bit more relaxed, less stressed, or more comfortable in doing an activity that has been challenging in the past. Changes of this sort are the beginning of generating a positive rather than negative feedback loop, so that greater ease in movement leads to a little less pain, less distress, more energy, and better sleep.

Over the course of the next six weeks or so, as you make your way through this book and develop more familiarity with the practices, we expect you'll gradually experience more and more pain relief, ease, joy, and peace of mind. The following anecdote illustrates how these practices can have a clear effect on both how you utilize your attention and the pain itself.

Hank's Story

A large, burly man in his late-fifties, Hank had suffered a back injury working on an oil rig in Alaska. For more than a decade, he had experienced unremitting chronic pain, primarily in his back and hips, which eventually led to permanent disability. He had undergone several extensive spinal surgeries that actually made his pain worse, resulting in the diagnosis of "failed back syndrome."

A friend who had taken our Mindful Yoga course suggested he might find it helpful, and though skeptical, he reluctantly signed up. During the posture practice, Hank was following instructions for how to relate to all bodily sensations from a curious, accepting, nonreactive perspective. As he was going through a flowing movement, he suddenly was gripped by an intense cramp in his right thigh. We asked him to rest on his yoga mat for a few moments, and to bring his attention as best he could to the full range of sensations in his body—not just the pain, but also the feeling of his breath moving in and out, the temperature of the air in the room, and the points of contact between his body and the mat underneath.

We also asked him to notice that right at the center of his experience of each of these sensations was his simple sense of presence, simple being. As he held steady for a few breaths and sustained this patient and courageous way of observing his in-the-moment sensations, Hank noticed that the tightness in his right thigh muscles released and then the pain there disappeared. He also discovered that his back pain dropped to a level that was much easier to tolerate. He was able to resume the posture practice and then do the meditation practice for the first time.

The following week, Hank shared that when practicing postures at home he again noticed a pattern of muscles suddenly tensing and becoming painful. At such times he was again able to pause and spread out his attention to notice other sensations and also simple being, and the tension would subside. He said, "Gradually over the week my back pain has gotten better. I'm feeling more confident that I can really do yoga!"

Mindful Yoga Practices

Meditation

Meditation has been practiced for its uplifting effects for more than five thousand years. The earliest archaeological evidence of meditation dates to around 3500 BC, in the Indus River Valley area of India. Over the millennia, the practice of meditation gradually spread to Europe in the West and as far as Japan in the East. Today, meditation is practiced all over the world.

Traditionally, the goals of meditation practice have been to achieve enduring happiness and gain freedom from suffering, through insight into our deepest nature. More recent, the health benefits of meditation have drawn many people to its practice. The past several decades have witnessed an impressive tide of research documenting substantial benefits from the practice of meditation (Baer 2003; Carlson and Garland 2005; Carson et al. 2004; Epel et al. 2009; Smith et al. 2005; Vollestad, Nielsen, and Nielsen 2012). Evidence now suggests that regular meditation practice is associated with improvements in a wide variety of conditions, including the following partial list:

Chronic pain	Premenstrual syndrome symptoms
Depression	Menopausal symptoms
Anxiety disorders	Sexual dysfunction
Stress levels	Immune function
Fatigue	Cortisol levels
Insomnia	Overall quality of life
Cardiovascular disease	Aging process (cellular telomerase activity)
Diabetes management	
Epilepsy	Blood pressure
Asthma	Working memory and test scores
Psoriasis	Relaxation ability
Hypertension	Vigor
Irritable bowel syndrome	Relationship satisfaction in couples
Substance abuse	Psychological well-being
Eating disorders	Attention and concentration
	Cancer recovery

The most recent studies of meditation often include tracking changes in brain structure and function. Neuroplastic changes have been documented in numerous brain regions that are crucial to attention regulation, emotion regulation (especially calming fear), and body awareness (Davidson et al. 2003; Grant 2014; Holzel et al. 2011; Holzel et al. 2007).

There are many different types of meditation with somewhat differing effects. An important initial process with nearly all forms of meditation is to develop some stability in how we use our attention by focusing on one or more "anchor points." In mindfulness meditation, the anchors are aspects of present-moment experience—in other words, whatever can be reliably noticed in the present moment. Usually, these anchors are the breath, whatever sounds arise, and whatever sensations are felt. So rather than focusing on something imaginary (like a golden light or a flowing brook), mindfulness meditation brings attention to what is already part of your direct experience here and now. The meditation practice you will begin this week—Breath and Simple Being—uses breath and simple being as anchor points.

A common discovery among beginning meditators (and even experienced meditators) is that it doesn't take long before your attention wanders off, kind of like a restless puppy. Your attention may get pulled into a thought, a sensation, an emotional feeling, or something else arising from your environment. This is perfectly natural. Our nervous system is conditioned to pay attention to whatever is most noticeable or seems important.

For example, you may be driving at night listening to music and then you hear the sound of a car horn. Your attention, in that moment, will likely move from the music to the horn because your nervous system perceives it to be important. The horn might be important—for instance, because someone is trying to alert you that your headlights are off. But the horn could just as easily be *not* important for you, as when someone is honking a greeting to a friend on the sidewalk.

Remember, it is natural (and unavoidable) for attention to be drawn away from a point of focus. When you realize that that has happened, first notice the direction your attention was pulled. Was your attention drawn toward a thought, a sensation, or something else? Then gently return your attention to the anchor point. Every time you notice attention being drawn away and practice returning to the anchor point, your ability to stabilize your attention strengthens. In other words, meditation is training your mind and helping "rewire" your brain in a healthier manner.

> **Practice noticing where your attention has been drawn, and then practice returning your attention to the anchor point.**

Before beginning the Breath and Simple Being meditation as indicated below, please explore the following two brief exercises for discovering simple being.

"I Am"

Notice that the word "I" is our common way of referring to our essential nature, simple being. This most intimate aspect of yourself that you call "I" is always present in any situation, at any given moment, and is always the same, no matter what changes have taken place in or around you.

Note that an audio recording of this exercise is also available at http://www. newharbinger.com/43287.

When you have a few minutes free and are by yourself, close your eyes and entertain this thought: "I am a person who _____" and just see all the descriptors your mind comes up with to fill in the blank. Most likely your mind will readily provide numerous descriptions of various aspects of your experience, such as your likes and dislikes, the roles you have had, and so forth.

After a few minutes of this, turn your attention to how you're *feeling* at the moment, and notice how those various self-defining thoughts leave you feeling.

Next, let those various mental descriptions fade away. In their place, stay with the simple sense: "I am." Not "I am this or that," but just "I *am*." For a minute or so, rest into the sense: "I am, I am, I am…"

After another minute or so, again notice how you're feeling. What is the resonance that this simple statement "I am" leaves you with?

If your experience is like that of most people, you will find that focusing on "I am" brings with it a feeling of simplicity, clarity, steadiness, and relative calm. In contrast, your mind's various descriptions of you may bring forth all sorts of other feelings, such as proud, anxious, uncertain, and the like. Often these feelings will not reflect calm, clarity, steadiness, or simplicity.

Simple Being, Always Here

For this exercise, please follow the instructions for the "Simple Being, Always Here" audio recording available at http://www.newharbinger.com/43287.

Week 2 Recommended Practice Schedule

Formal Practice

Record notes on the formal practice calendar. Jot down your practice times and observations on the weekly calendar provided at the end of this chapter.

Postures

Week 2 Yoga Posture Sequence. Turn to the "Mindful Yoga Posture Practices" section on page 133 and follow the instructions for Week 2; you can also follow along with the downloadable video available at http://www.newharbinger.com/43287. Practice every other day, at least three times this week. As you do the postures, simply notice waves of various bodily sensations: stretching, holding, releasing, tingling, and so on.

Breathing

Three-Part Breath. Practice each day (with or without the downloadable audio at http://www.newharbinger.com/43287).

Meditation

Breath and Simple Being. Use the recording at http://www.newharbinger.com/43287, and practice at least five times this week.

Informal Practice

Self-study. Spend a few moments each day discovering how your attention functions by focusing on various types of experience: touch, sounds, sights, smells, tastes. Try to refrain from attempting to change or "fix" any of the sensations—discover what it's like to just notice their presence. Reconnect with simple being, just noticing that you are present, as you feel whatever else is present.

Keeping the company of truth. On the following worksheet, describe what you have observed and learned about how attention functions.

Keeping the Company of Truth: Riding the Waves of Attention

Spend a few moments each day directing your attention to the arising, cresting, and subsiding of various types of sensations: touch (e.g., warmth or coolness, rough or smooth), sights, sounds, smells, tastes—and also briefly reconnecting with Simple Being at that time.	Did directing your attention to these wave-like patterns, and reconnecting with Simple Being seem to make any difference? If so, please briefly describe.
Day 1	
Day 2	
Day 3	
Day 4	
Day 5	
Day 6	
Day 7	

Week 2 Formal Practice—Riding the Waves of Attention

Record time spent in each practice. Note any observations.

	Breath Three-Part Breath	Meditation Breath and Simple Being	Postures Week 2		Observations What did you notice about waves of attention and waves of sensations during your formal practice?
Day 1 Time					
Notes					
Day 2 Time					
Notes					
Day 3 Time					
Notes					

	Breath Three-Part Breath	Meditation Breath and Simple Being	Postures Week 2	Observations What did you notice about waves of attention and waves of sensations during your formal practice?
Day 4 Time				
Notes				
Day 5 Time				
Notes				
Day 6 Time				
Notes				
Day 7 Time				
Notes				

Week 2 Review

Before going further, let's review what you have learned from Week 2.

First, practice the Breath and Simple Being audio-guided meditation at http://www .newharbinger.com/43287.

Next, briefly look over Week 2 and ask yourself, "Why is learning to use attention skillfully so important?" Review the "Week 2 Recommended Practice Schedule."

Did you follow through on your commitment to practice the breath, postures, and meditation as suggested?

_____

_____

What did you notice before, during, and after your practices?

_____

_____

How would you describe any changes in your experience that you may have detected?

_____

_____

Did you notice any agitation or impatience?

_____

_____

What have you noticed about your pain?

_____

_____

Describe how your Mindful Yoga practices have affected you this week.

_____

_____

_____

You may still be finding it challenging to practice regularly. And you also may be having expectations that didn't match your experience, such as "I need to empty my mind" or "It must be quiet so I can meditate." Here are a few common concerns and our suggestions for addressing them:

I'm having difficulty finding a regular practice rhythm.

Be patient if you weren't able to follow a regular schedule—it's important to keep trying. It may take several weeks to find a practice rhythm that works for you. Remember that some practice is better than no practice. Notice any resistance that arises when you try to engage in this self-care routine. Become curious about what is driving this resistance.

I can't quiet my mind.

It's a common misconception that meditation requires emptying the mind. In fact, meditation involves refining how you use your attention. And if we expect total silence to meditate, we'll never even start! Expectations like these can get in the way of what's really happening during meditation.

It can be useful, as you begin meditation, to set an intention to simply do your best to stay connected with the anchor points that are the focus of your meditation. For now, this will be your breath and your feeling of being present. Then, each time you discover that your attention has wandered—which happens even to experienced meditators—just notice without judgment that your attention has wandered, and then bring your focus back to your anchor.

You might simply think to yourself, "Ah, attention has wandered." Then reorient your attention with a gentle effort, as if guiding the hand of a small child, without fully engaging with your thoughts. Just begin to notice your breath, or simple being, again. Over time, you'll gradually find that your attention is becoming more stable.

You'll also find that your attention is more flexible—"noises" that seemed so distracting before are no longer so captivating, and you can just let them be, you don't have to push them away. With more practice, you will discover that this steadiness and flexibility of attention is critical for skillfully navigating daily life.

My mind is too busy to meditate!

Although somewhat surprising and unexpected, there are valuable discoveries to be made *every time* your attention wanders. You will begin to understand more clearly what attracts your attention—what types of thoughts, emotions, and sensations are vying for attention. These insights can help in steering yourself toward relief and resiliency.

For example, you may discover that habits of thought, like "This stinks and it'll never change," often arise when your pain gets bad. Some of these habitual thoughts can potentially make your pain worse. As we'll explore later in this book, being able to clearly see these habits will allow for different ways of viewing your experience.

In addition to recognizing the patterns at play in your mind and in your emotions, every time you return your attention to the object of meditation, your brain gets a bit stronger at returning. This is not unlike building physical strength. Every time you flex a muscle, it gets stronger and more agile. Likewise, every time you refocus your attention in meditation, your brain is strengthening its healthy responses.

WEEK 3

Riding the Waves of Stress

With the boat of Simple Being a wise person crosses over the threatening ocean currents.

—Svetasvatara Upanishad (yogic text, c. 400 BC)

In our fast-paced world—filled with financial pressures, health challenges, political unrest, and weather extremes—most people struggle with stress. In fact, 80 percent of adults say they experience at least one symptom of stress, such as headache and/or feeling overwhelmed, anxious, or depressed (American Psychological Association 2017).

Of course, pain itself is stressful. And, unfortunately, the relationship between stress and pain is reciprocal: *Chronic stress is a primary culprit in the onset of chronic pain.* The result is a vicious cycle: Stress can exacerbate pain, and pain can exacerbate stress.

Clearly, learning more skillful ways to reduce stress is essential to enhancing health. The first step is to understand what makes something stressful in the first place.

Imagine the following scenario: You're snug in bed, drifting off to sleep, when you hear a noise outside. Your mind starts racing with the idea that a burglar is trying to break into your home. Your heart begins to pound and your breath quickens as you feel a sense of mounting panic—should you call 911? Your muscles tense, your pain sharply intensifies, and your stomach tightens as you agonize about your situation. You stumble out of bed, pull on your bathrobe, go to the door, and listen. Hearing no other sounds outside, you crack the door and peak out. Seeing nothing unusual, you go outside, walk around your house, still finding nothing. Finally you go back to bed, but end up tossing and turning for hours.

Now imagine an alternate scenario: You're snug in bed, drifting off to sleep, when you hear a noise outside. You try to remember whether you put the lid on the trash can and wonder if raccoons have knocked it over. You

> **Stress can exacerbate pain, and pain can exacerbate stress.**

consider getting up and turning on the light to see what's going on, but decide that you'll deal with any mess in the morning. You roll over and go back to sleep.

The same event—hearing a bump in the night—can result in a completely different set of immediate reactions, depending on your mind's interpretation of what's happening. If you tell yourself, "It's a burglar!" you are thrust into panic mode, you become tense, your pain gets worse, and you have a hard time getting back to sleep. Plus, the next day would almost certainly be one of those "bad days" when you're exhausted, easily irritated, and dealing with a pain flare. But if you tell yourself, "That rascally raccoon!" the noise is a momentary bother that wakes you up, but soon you are sound asleep—and the next day is a regular one during which you may not even remember to check whether your trash can got knocked over.

The point of comparing these two scenarios is to clarify the essence of stress: *It's all a matter of perception. Stress is defined as any perception of threat to our interests, together with feeling unable to cope adequately* (Lazarus and Folkman 1984). Life inevitably entails many challenging situations, some minor and some major. "Stressors"—that is, the initial triggers for stress—may be external events, such as being cut off in traffic, arguments, or uncertainty at work; or internal events, such as physical discomfort, worrisome thoughts, or unsettling emotions. Regardless of whether the trigger is external or internal, events become stressors depending on how you perceive and react to them.

Whenever your mind interprets an event to be potentially difficult or even harmful, your fight-or-flight stress reaction kicks in automatically. Your body prepares for an emergency by speeding up your breath and heart rate, and tensing your muscles. Typically, your mind will also start racing.

It's critical to recognize that the story your mind spins about a situation often can make your stress reaction worse. Any assumptions, hopes, and fears you have—for example, "I'm no match for a burglar" or "I'm always so unlucky"—can set up expectations that may not be rooted in reality and needlessly fuel your stress reaction. Although some degree of discouraging thoughts may be inevitable, buying into and dwelling on such thoughts is like pouring gasoline on a fire. The idea here is not to pretend that threats don't exist but to recognize the importance of learning to respond appropriately to a potential stressor—to make well-informed and healthy choices that are grounded in the reality of the present situation rather than to react mindlessly out of habit.

Any time you're dealing with a stressful moment, it's especially crucial to pay close attention to how things unfold—in particular, noticing the stories your mind tells about the situation and observing any emotions, sensations, and additional thoughts that may arise. When you're stressed, the ways you react and the decisions you make can have a big impact on many aspects of your life, including your pain and fatigue levels, mood, mental clarity, and the overall outcome of the situation. By paying close attention when you're under stress, you can learn to recognize the physical, emotional, and mental reactions that habitually tend to overtake you—and then you can discover healthier ways to respond to life's challenges.

Riding vs. Battling the Waves of Stress

Just like everything in life—for example, sound waves, heartbeats, and pain—stress reactions occur in wavelike patterns. Stress begins, builds, peaks, and fades. The common tendency is to try to block or battle the waves of stress. Everyone knows this may work for a short while, but over time, it is completely exhausting and futile.

Fortunately, there is another way. One of the first landmark meditation investigations demonstrated that meditation can transform how we handle stress. At Harvard University, psychologists compared the stress reactions of experienced meditators to non-meditators while both groups were shown gory films of dramatic industrial accidents (Goleman and Schwartz 1976). Somewhat surprising, the meditators at first showed stronger stress reactions as measured by heart rate and skin arousal tests. However, their reactions settled back to normal much more quickly than the non-meditators. The meditators also reported lower anxiety.

This study illustrates two encouraging effects of regular meditation: First, meditation allows us to become *more aware and responsive*—rather than numb—to stress in the moment it arises. This is important, because stressful situations such as car accidents often call for a quick and powerful response. Second, once a stressful situation has passed, meditation permits us to rapidly return to a calmer state, so that we are ready to encounter whatever the next moment brings—whether that is something pleasant or the opposite.

One of the key skills that can be learned through mindfulness meditation is how to allow the arousal of the stress reaction to arise, peak, and subside—to let the wave wash through your system without trying to block it or change it. This skill supports both your responsiveness to stress as well as your ability to calm your system back to its baseline.

Since it's often not so much the stressor itself that creates problems but how we perceive and respond to it, over time we can learn to "ride the waves of stress" rather than continually battle them. For many of us, learning to notice our physical, mental, and emotional reactions to stress can be transformative. That's because most of us go through our lives completely unaware that our stress reactions have become an ingrained habit that tends to stick around for hours, causing physical tension and emotional distress. Not only does this tension and distress harm our health, it also strongly exacerbates pain and related problems such as fatigue. By becoming aware of these automatic stress reactions and learning how to respond to them effectively, we can develop more skillful ways of handling challenges and become more resilient when faced with difficulty.

Awareness of how you use your attention moment to moment is the key to making this critical shift from battling waves of stress to learning how to ride them. As you read through the next several paragraphs, please follow along with the corresponding sections of the Riding vs. Battling the Waves of Stress chart on the opposite page (Carson and Carson 2018).

How Stress Works

Stress starts with some event—external or internal—that you perceive as a threat (see top of chart). This perception triggers an immediate set of physiological and mental reactions that tend to feed on one another—the more physical tension you feel, the more your mind races, and the more difficult the situation appears. The key to whether this set of reactions continues to escalate or begins to settle is how well you are paying attention, how aware you are of these various reactions.

If you are not consciously attentive to your stress reactions, then you end up battling the waves (see left side of chart). An automatic pattern of habitual reactions unfolds, including feelings that are increasingly difficult, more pain, and other physical symptoms. Then you succumb to the negative spiraling of your mind's interpretation. Driven by these escalating reactions, the urge to act can prompt behaviors that ultimately backfire. This may include overreactions that tend to make things worse or struggling to make the stress go away, which leaves you more exhausted.

In the short term, stress continues to build, so that you're often feeling stressed out and experiencing more pain. Unfortunately, what you've just done is practice the stress reaction. We get good at what we practice, which means this same unhealthy stress reaction is more likely to happen again. Over the long term, stress is accelerated. This repeated cascade of battling the waves can lead to breakdown, both physical and psychological.

On the other hand, if you are consciously attentive to your initial stress reactions, then you can find your balance and ride the waves (see right side of chart). You can apply yoga practices—such as slowing your breathing—to help you stay present with feelings as they momentarily surge, with thoughts as they swirl, and with symptoms as they briefly ramp up. When you pay attention to your stress reactions, your urge to action is both attuned to what you are feeling and guided by awareness of your options. Your behavior can include skillful choices, such as clear communications, that allow you to effectively address the situation. In the short term, stress is reduced and calms down more quickly. This way of consciously working with stress leads to long-term personal growth in terms of insight into yourself and others, and becoming more resilient and compassionate about the struggles we all have with stress.

Coping with Stress: Riding vs. Battling the Waves

Events/Stressors
(external events, thoughts, feelings, bodily sensations)

Perception of Difficulty/Arousal Begins

Mental Reaction		**Physiological Reaction**
Thoughts race and your mind's story activates, including assumptions, hopes, fears, beliefs, and so on	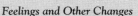	Muscles tighten, heart rate increases, breath quickens or shallows, blood pressure increases, adrenaline output rises, and so on

CONSCIOUSLY ATTENTIVE?	
Battling the Waves	*Riding the Waves*
Automatic and unconscious fight-or-flight response kicks in, and a habitual pattern of reacting unfolds.	An awareness of automatic reactions develops, leading to an ability to respond more effectively to events.
Feelings and Other Changes	
Difficult emotions (anger, sadness, fear) and physical symptoms (bodily pain, headaches, etc.) arise, and negative thoughts spiral.	Difficult feelings and physical symptoms arise, but briefly, allowing space to relax, breathe freely, get centered, and distinguish the event from the mind's story.
Urge to Action	
Strong emotions, discomfort in the body, and habitual negative thoughts drive the urge to react.	Awareness of emotions and physical symptoms allows recognition of options for responding.
Behavior	
Poor communication, withdrawal, striking out, suppression of feelings, overdoing, or substance abuse results.	Clearer communication, caregiving, mutual problem-solving, or healthy self-soothing results.
Short-Term Implications	
Stress persists: chronic hyperarousal, more pain, repetition of the stress reaction cycle.	Stress reduction: quicker recovery of mental equanimity and physical equilibrium, less pain.
Long-Term Implications	
Breakdown: physical/psychological exhaustion, increased chronic pain, anxiety, depression, susceptibility to illness, deterioration in relationships.	Growth: confidence in coping abilities, decreased chronic pain, greater understanding of self and others, capacity to help others cope, greater peace of mind.

Ultimately you realize that the only way to meet the challenge of stress is to stay with it and learn to ride these waves. Instead of trying to make stress go away, if you are willing to stay with it, you gain direct insight into how stress is whipped up and perpetuated by getting caught up in your mind's swirling thoughts and emotional reactions. Once you see this clearly, you can learn not to buy into—that is, not take literally—the stories your mind weaves. As a result, the whole stress cascade can unfold much more favorably.

> **Becoming better at coping with stress can itself help relieve stress.**

An added bonus is that becoming better at coping with stress can itself help relieve stress. Remember, getting stressed involves *feeling unable to cope adequately with a stressor*. So when your confidence in your ability to cope strengthens, that itself can dampen stress reactions. Likewise, you will eventually begin to perceive fewer events as threats. For example, the exhausted and short-tempered clerk at the market is no longer seen as a personal threat.

The Mindful Yoga practices offer an ideal laboratory for practicing riding the waves of stress. Yoga postures often put us in challenging positions, for example, balancing on one leg, which gives us the opportunity to notice any thoughts, accompanying emotions, and physical sensations that arise from this challenge.

Practicing awareness of stress reactions during movement, such as fear or frustration, allows us to observe these tendencies "in action." Noticing—yet remaining nonreactive—to these small stress reactions in response to movement supports the body in finding ease as it returns to healthy, functional movement.

During meditation, all kinds of thoughts can arise. For example, you might think, "Am I doing this right or just wasting my time?" These thoughts are typically accompanied by related emotions and sensations. This week, when doing the yoga practices, see if you can refrain from trying to "fix" or judge yourself for experiencing these stress reactions. Instead, do your best to just be curious about your stress habits—observe how they arise and operate in the moment. Later, as we continue our voyage toward resiliency and pain relief, we will apply particular skills to working with stress reactions.

Jerry's Story

Jerry loved being outdoors, and his work as a cable installation technician allowed him to spend much of each workday outside. He was also an avid sportsman, enjoying fishing, golf, and other sports that landed him in nature. However, in his midforties after a bad car accident, he spent six weeks in the hospital followed by four months in a rehab center. A year later, even though his injuries had mostly healed, he continued to have severe pain in his neck and spine. The pain made it impossible for Jerry to resume the work and outdoor sports that he enjoyed. He found a part-time desk job, but soon was caught in a dark spell, quite depressed about his losses. His physical therapist suggested he sign up for our Mindful Yoga course.

During the third class, as Jerry was practicing the gentle yoga movements, he suddenly felt his whole body tense up.

"I'm stuck, and it really hurts!" he exclaimed.

The teacher asked, "What would it be like to just stay with what you're feeling, for a few moments?"

"I can't," he said, "plus now my heart is racing!"

The teacher asked what else he noticed. As Jerry got more curious about what he was actually experiencing, he discovered that he was afraid he was going to hurt himself. Jerry noticed his thoughts had latched on to what had happened several months before, when he had tried to reengage in regular exercise but ended up overexerting himself and just hurting more. He could see at that moment that his body was tensing up during the yoga class to protect itself from what his mind was projecting—and that's why he was experiencing such strong physical and emotional reactions.

As Jerry got clear that the gentle yoga postures were not what he was reacting to, his muscles began to release, his pain lessened, and his heartbeat returned to a normal pace. He was able to reengage in the class, and at the end of the final relaxation pose, he felt calm and more at ease. And he knew he had discovered a very important lesson about learning to ride his waves of stress.

Week 3 Recommended Practice Schedule

Formal Practice

Record notes on the formal practice calendar. Jot down your practice times and observations on the weekly calendar provided at the end of this chapter.

Postures

Week 3 Yoga Posture Sequence. Turn to the "Mindful Yoga Posture Practices" section on page 133 and follow the instructions for Week 3; you can also follow along with the downloadable video available at http://www.newharbinger.com/43287. Practice every other day, at least three times this week. As you do the postures, simply notice any waves of stress (arising, cresting, and settling), and without trying to "fix" stress, see what you can discover about these waves.

Breathing

Three-Part Breath. Practice each day (with or without the downloadable audio at http://www.newharbinger.com/43287).

Meditation

Breath and Simple Being. Use the recording at http://www.newharbinger.com/43287, and practice at least five times this week.

Informal Practice

Self-study. Become curious about the waves of stress—the physical, emotional, and cognitive waves. Refrain from trying to "fix" or judge yourself for experiencing these stress reactions. Reconnect with simple being, just noticing you are present, even in the midst of stress.

Keeping the company of truth. On the following worksheet, describe what you have observed and learned about stress.

Keeping the Company of Truth: Riding the Waves of Stress

When feeling stressed in your daily life, see if you can notice some of the stress waves passing through—such as quicker breathing or muscles tightening. Also try to briefly reconnect with simple being at that time.	Did watching the waves of stress and reconnecting with simple being seem to make any difference? If so, briefly describe.
Day 1	
Day 2	
Day 3	
Day 4	
Day 5	
Day 6	
Day 7	

Week 3 Formal Practice—Riding the Waves of Stress

Record time spent in each practice. Note any observations.

	Breath Three-Part Breath	Meditation Breath and Simple Being	Postures Week 3	Observations What did you notice about waves of stress during your formal practice?
Day 1 Time				
Notes				
Day 2 Time				
Notes				
Day 3 Time				
Notes				

	Breath Three-Part Breath	Meditation Breath and Simple Being	Postures Week 3	Observations What did you notice about waves of stress during your formal practice?
Day 4 Time				
Notes				
Day 5 Time				
Notes				
Day 6 Time				
Notes				
Day 7 Time				
Notes				

Week 3 Review

Before going further, let's review what you have learned in Week 3.

First, practice the Breath and Simple Being audio-guided meditation.

Next, look back over Week 3 and ask yourself:

What did I discover about stress?

_____

_____

Did I become aware of my stress reaction earlier than usual?

_____

_____

Were there moments when I could simply observe my own stress response?

_____

_____

How did stress impact my pain levels?

_____

_____

Summarize how your formal and informal practices affected you.

_____

_____

_____

Remember, most people experience obstacles while learning these new skills and while trying to fit the practices into their busy lives. It's perfectly normal to find these practices challenging. Sometimes it may even feel as if stress levels are increasing—not only because the practices take up time but also because recognizing your habits of reactivity can be unsettling.

However, the research, along with our experience with thousands of people, indicates that doing the practices is the key to building your personal bridge to relief and resilience. So please just do your best. Keep in mind the important foundational practice of love—that is, *be kind and loving toward yourself*—when working with the stress of establishing a yoga practice.

Here are some common challenges you might be facing, along with how to address them:

I'm trying to stay present with stress, but it's just getting worse.

This is a very common complaint. Many of us would prefer to ignore stress rather than draw attention to it. A strong human tendency is to pull things we like toward us and push away or ignore things we don't like. But turning away from stress blinds us to the truth of what's happening in our body, heart, and mind. In the Mindful Yoga approach, we practice staying present with stress and observing what is true in any given moment. This develops our ability to recognize what is really going on in less obvious aspects of ourselves: physically, emotionally, and mentally. Staying present is the only way we can become aware of habits we have developed that may be harmful. Stick with it and see what happens!

This is stressful!

Finding time to practice can be a strain, plus it's hard to learn any new skill—whether it's playing the guitar or meditating. There are times when practicing feels frustrating and even painful. Yet the rewards can be profound, including enhanced functioning and brighter mood—and sometimes it can even *add* time to your life, in terms of better sleep and giving you more time for your favorite activities, and a longer lifespan (meditation has been shown to slow the aging process) (Epel et al. 2009). That's why it's essential to commit to the practice and remain patient as you build stamina. Whatever you practice, you gradually get better at it, and that makes it easier and more rewarding. And for many of us, the practice eventually becomes an enjoyable part of our day.

WEEK 4

Riding the Waves of the Mind's Story

Feeling bound or free depends only upon the mind.

—Amritabindu Upanishad (yogic text, c. 400 BC)

Our minds are powerful and our thoughts shape our reality—which is important to recognize when it comes to the experience of chronic pain. In a now-famous experiment, college students were fitted with a helmet that they were told was an Electric Stimulator that would deliver a shock to their skulls (Bayer, Baer, and Early 1991). As the experimenter turned a knob, the students could see an intensity meter display a rising electric current. The higher it climbed, the more pain the students reported experiencing. However, the helmet was a modified old hair dryer that didn't deliver any electric shock at all.

This experiment *doesn't* mean that the students weren't experiencing "real pain." Rather, this and similar experiments demonstrate that, when your mind is convinced something will be painful, your brain will react by generating pain. As the saying goes: *"The mind is a wonderful servant but a terrible master."*

The process by which our minds are shaping and filtering our experiences is going on all the time, 24/7, and is by no means restricted to situations that appear potentially harmful. To make this clear, we invite you to engage in another experiment—but one that won't hurt at all. Please spend a minute or two gazing at the image on the next page. As you do this, notice what comes to mind. Does the picture remind you of somewhere or something you've seen or experienced?

> **"The mind is a wonderful servant but a terrible master."**

Perhaps it evokes a particular emotion, thought, or dream. Write down a few words describing whatever ideas or images come to mind as you look at this picture.

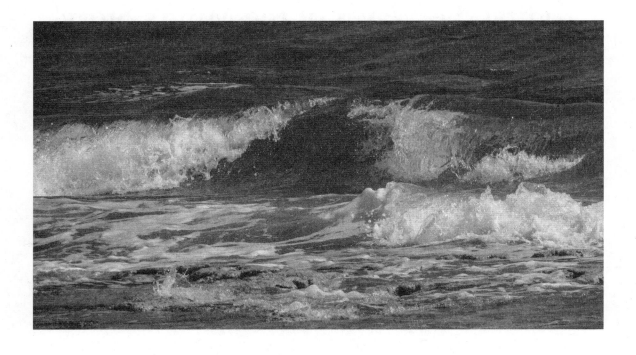

_____

_____

_____

_____

_____

We've done this same experiment—viewing a picture of ocean waves and seeing what comes to mind—countless times with many different people. What we've found is that the same image tends to elicit a wide variety of responses. Some people say it makes them feel calm, while others report the opposite—that it makes them feel agitated. Some are reminded of fun times at the beach, while others recall a frightening time when they themselves or someone they knew almost drowned.

The main point of this experiment, in combination with the "shock helmet" experiment described above, is this: *Our minds make associations nearly all the time between whatever we perceive at a given moment and what we have experienced in the past or imagine we may experience in the future.* These associations often get woven into a mental narrative or "story"— that is, our minds try to make sense of what we perceive by connecting perceptions with associated thoughts, memories, feelings, and mental images. And our minds do this continually, regardless of whether an event is pleasant, difficult, or neutral—or whether it happens to us or to someone else. The stories woven by different minds can vary greatly, depending on our cultural backgrounds, personalities, and past—for example, whether we love the ocean or fear it.

There are at least two reasons why our minds are continually weaving stories. First, our minds are attempting to prepare us for whatever may come next—despite the fact that, in reality, the future always remains unknown. Second, our minds are naturally very imaginative and creative. Were it not for this imaginative ability, we would not have all the books, movies, music, art, and other forms of creative expression that enrich our lives.

But just as the themes in books and movies can be tragic or benevolent or comical, so too can the stories your mind weaves be threatening or sad, inspiring or joyful. And to the extent that you've become accustomed to experiencing the world through the filter of your mind's narratives, these mental stories impact you—they can provoke not only emotional suffering but physiological pain as well. When you "fuse" with—that is, buy into or get lost in—your mind's stories, you are likely to become swept up by all kinds of anticipations, accompanied by emotional and physiological ups and downs, and may lose sight of the actual reality of your situation.

For this reason it's crucial to distinguish between an event, pure and simple, and the stories your mind weaves about that event. To understand this more clearly, let's return to the photo of the wave. The picture you see is identical in the thousands of copies of this book. But what you wrote about the picture is unique. Your mind's associations with the photo are entirely personal—memories, interpretations, and feelings that correspond to you and might not reflect someone else's narrative. Can you recognize that these associated experiences, this "story" your mind wove when looking at the photo, is not the same as the photo itself nor is it contained in the photo?

Let's try another brief experiment. Return to looking at the image for a minute or so, but this time, find out if you can—at least for a few moments—stay with just seeing the picture as it is, without engaging with mental labels, comments, or associations that may arise. When you attempt this, don't try to *stop* thoughts or feelings from coming forth—just focus as clearly as you can on what your eyes are actually seeing in the photo itself. Continue reading below after you have done this experiment.

Were you able to sidestep mental commentary about the picture for a few moments? If so, you were experiencing what meditation teachers refer to as *bare attention*. Even if you were not able to experience bare attention, hopefully you were able to recognize that the content of the photo—for example, the foam on the waves, the curl of the surf—is distinct from your mental interpretations *about* the photo. This is key: Thoughts are always *about* something, but thoughts never *are* that something itself, any more than your thoughts about your favorite food are the same as tasting that food in your mouth.

> **Thoughts are always *about* something, but thoughts never *are* that something itself.**

Fusion Leads to Confusion

Learning to recognize when we fuse with the mind's story—that is, when we mistake what the mind is projecting onto an event as the reality of the event itself—is a valuable skill. Our mind's stories are made up mostly of either thoughts, images, and memories about the past, or expectations and imaginations about the unknown future. However, life is always unfolding right now; life never happens in the past or future. As we strengthen our ability to see when fusion is happening, we can avoid confusing our mind's story with what is actually present. When we can pay attention to what is really happening, here and now, then our decisions can be guided by what we clearly notice, rather than getting mixed up with our mind's stories about the situation.

Remember that a major driving force in any stress reaction is how your mind interprets events. So if you need to make an important decision but are fused with your mind's story, then that story—which may not reflect reality—largely dictates your reactions.

For example, recall the "bump in the night" scenarios from the previous chapter. Neurological research makes clear that our brain responds to a real event and an imagined story about the event in a very similar manner. In either case, the same processes are triggered in our body. If we hear a noise outside our window at night and immediately fuse with—that is, buy into—the thought that the "bump" is the sound of a burglar, then "fusion leads to confusion" and we experience a full set of stress reactions: racing thoughts, shallow breathing, flaring pain, feeling alarmed, and so forth. Typically, confusion then leads to poor decisions—for example, setting off your car alarm to scare the suspected prowler and disturbing the entire neighborhood, rather than attempting to verify what really caused the noise.

By clearly distinguishing between events and the mind's stories about events—what we call "riding the waves of the mind's story"—we can refrain from assuming the next moment will be a repeat of a past moment and make better, more clearly informed decisions about how to handle whatever challenges arise. To stay clear-headed and focus on "just the facts" takes practice. Otherwise, we're likely to fall into a trap of our own making, which is where Jane ended up for a long time.

Jane's Story

Jane loved riding her Harley. Raised in the Northwest, at eighteen she was president of her high school's motorcycle club, leading long weekend rides along winding roads with stunning views of the Cascade mountains. After graduation, she enlisted in the army, following in the footsteps of her grandfather and father, who had both seen action during their tours of duty. Jane trained as a medic and served as a sergeant during Desert Storm, directing a helicopter-based team that rescued wounded soldiers from the battlefield.

By the time she was discharged, Jane had suffered multiple back injuries from lifting litters onto helicopters. She used the GI Bill to become a physician assistant with the goal of helping fellow veterans at the local VA medical center. Drawing on her personal experience of the pain and loss that many vets endure, she became known as a very caring yet tough-love medical provider, helping many individuals cope with their injuries. She herself continued nonetheless to suffer from chronic pain, with her neck and back pain spreading until she was eventually diagnosed with fibromyalgia.

When Jane first came to Mindful Yoga, twenty-five years after leaving the army, she felt very limited in what she could do because she feared increased pain. Not only had she not ridden a motorcycle for twenty years, she hadn't gone dancing—another activity she used to love—for more than a decade. She also avoided doing yard work and refrained from walking more than a short distance. She said, "I'm injured, and I have no choice. These activities I love would only cause me more pain."

Driven by her mind's story, Jane became increasingly trapped by kinesiophobia—fear of movement—which is a primary factor contributing to disability among people with chronic pain (Roelofs et al. 2011). But the more she avoided activities, the more deconditioned her body became, to the point where almost anything she did left her feeling sore and achy. Her mind's story was amplified by fears predicting an eventual catastrophe: "I can't seem to do anything anymore! I'm afraid I'll become crippled and have to quit my job. There is no hope for me."

Jane was initially very skeptical about Mindful Yoga; she thought it was "too woo-woo" for her very pragmatic approach to life, but she enrolled anyway because of the persistent urging of a friend. To her total surprise, as she learned to observe and ride—rather than fuse with—her mind's fearful stories about heightened pain, she was able to comfortably do nearly all the yoga postures. Soon she found herself pain-free for the first time in twenty-five years.

"I'm completely amazed!" she shared in class, "I had no idea that my ideas about pain and what I couldn't do had affected me so much!" She gradually opened up to engaging in many activities that she had been avoiding. She discovered that, although she could certainly ramp up her pain if she overdid an activity, when she was moderate in her efforts she could do so much more—including weekend motorcycle rides with her husband and friends.

Here are some key points about riding the waves of the mind's story:

Our minds are generating stories, wave after wave, nearly all the time. When we fuse the mental stories and the real events together, it's similar to not noticing our eyeglasses because they are so close to our eyes—and if our glasses are tinted either gray or pink, everything we look at will also appear to take on that color. So, for example, if we believe that some activity will worsen our pain, we are likely to avoid it unquestioningly.

With practice, we can become aware of our mind's stories in all kinds of circumstances. Then, when we are dealing with challenging situations, the skill of distinguishing between events and our mind's stories can help us avoid getting caught up in the mind's powerful momentum. We end up feeling clearer and calmer, and make better choices, including about how to handle situations that impact chronic pain. We can ride the waves of whatever is happening without getting knocked down.

Love and acceptance are very relevant to this skill. As you learn to observe your mind generating stories, you may find it surprising to discover that your mind is always so busy trying to figure everything out. Once you become aware of your mind's many imaginative stories, a tendency to judge yourself can take hold, to put yourself down for having these thoughts—labeling them "silly" or "stupid." But rather than judge your mind, kindly remember that your mind is just trying to protect you, just trying to be a good problem solver—even though these mental efforts sometimes add to the problem and make pain more limiting rather than less so.

Week 4 Recommended Practice Schedule

Formal Practice

Record notes on the formal practice calendar. Jot down your practice times and observations on the weekly calendar at the end of this chapter.

Postures

Week 4 Yoga Posture Sequence. Turn to the "Mindful Yoga Posture Practices" section on page 133 and follow the instructions for Week 4; you can also follow along with the downloadable video available at http://www.newharbinger.com/43287. Practice every other day, at least three times this week. As you do the postures, from time to time tune in to your mind's inner dialogue and notice that your mind's commentary on the posture practice is distinct from your actual engagement in the postures. It might be easiest to bring attention to the mind's story between completing one posture and starting the next posture.

Breathing

Three-Part Breath. Practice each day (with or without the downloadable audio at http://www.newharbinger.com/43287).

Meditation

Breath Through Sensing. While continuing to build stability for attention, this meditation will also include flexibility in how you direct your attention. Use the audio recording at http://www.newharbinger.com/43287. Try it at least five times this week. This recording will extend your meditation practice. You will first attend to one aspect of experience—just breathing—for a while and then rest into simple being. Then you will be guided to notice any sounds that are arising in and around you, then back to simple being. Finally, you will be guided to notice various sensations present in your physical body, then back to simple being. Please take note of when your mind's story activates and begins to weave tales about the breath, the sounds, or the sensations. When that happens—and it will, over and over—each time notice that it happened and gently release your attention from your mind's story. Then redirect attention back to the aspect (breath, sound, sensation) you had been observing.

Informal Practice

Self-study. Spend a few moments each day observing your mind's story. Refrain from trying to fix or judge yourself for experiencing whatever you are experiencing. Become curious about these waves of thought patterns. How does your mind's story respond to, or have an effect on, your experience of various sounds, physical sensations, or mood states? Mental tendencies you might notice include:

- How an experience gets labeled and whether the label involves judgment. For example, is the sound of a garbage truck labeled as irritating?

- Does a particular experience get associated with another experience? For example, does getting stuck in traffic remind you of a past painful event that happened in traffic?

- Is there anticipation of what is coming? For example, if you have an appointment with a pain specialist, does your mind weave a story ahead of time about what's going to happen during the appointment?

Keeping the company of truth. On the following worksheet, describe what you have observed and learned about your mind's story.

Keeping the Company of Truth: Riding the Waves of the Mind's Story

Spend a few moments each day noticing the difference between the actual events you are witnessing and the stories your mind weaves about the events. Try doing this under various circumstances—some easy, others stressful. Also briefly reconnect with simple being at that time.	Did observing your mind's story and reconnecting with simple being seem to make any difference? If so, describe the event, what your mind's story was, and how this process of noticing affected you.
Day 1	
Day 2	
Day 3	
Day 4	
Day 5	
Day 6	
Day 7	

Week 4 Formal Practice—Riding the Waves of the Mind's Story

Record time spent in each practice. Note any observations.

	Breath Three-Part Breath	Meditation Breath Through Sensing	Postures Week 4	Observations What did you notice about the mind's story during your formal practice?
Day 1 Time				
Notes				
Day 2 Time				
Notes				
Day 3 Time				
Notes				

	Breath Three-Part Breath	Meditation Breath Through Sensing	Postures Week 4	Observations What did you notice about the mind's story during your formal practice?
Day 4 Time				
Notes				
Day 5 Time				
Notes				
Day 6 Time				
Notes				
Day 7 Time				
Notes				

Week 4 Review

Before going further, let's review what you have learned so far.

First, practice the Breath Through Sensing guided meditation available at http://www.newharbinger.com/43287.

Next, briefly review your practice and observations from Week 4.

Were you able to listen inward sometimes and ride the waves of the mind's story by recognizing that events—and what your mind has to say about them—are related but not the same thing?

_____

_____

Were you able to apply this skill while doing the yoga postures or during meditation?

_____

_____

How was meditation overall for you this week, with the extension of focusing on sounds and physical sensations?

_____

_____

Summarize how your formal and informal practices affected you this week.

_____

_____

_____

You are now halfway through the Mindful Yoga program. You've been introduced to the essential yoga practices and foundations, and have explored them to some extent. Hopefully, you are beginning to notice some positive changes in how you feel and function in daily life. In Weeks 5 through 7, these practices and foundations will be applied to specific symptoms that are especially problematic for people who live with chronic pain—pain itself, emotional changes, and fatigue.

Please take stock of what you have learned so far. Answer these key questions:

How is your formal practice going?

Are you having more success fitting in meditation, breathing, and posture practices now than during Week 1? If you haven't practiced as much as you'd like, what's been getting in your way? Considering that the research shows that more practice brings more benefit, is there anything you can do to fit in more practice? Even 10- or 15-minute sessions can have profound effects.

_____

_____

_____

Are you discovering anything new in the informal practices?

What have you learned from riding the waves of breath, stress, and the mind's story? Perhaps you're finding that there are stuck patterns that repeat themselves when you're feeling stressed, or when you tend to fuse with—and become confused by—the mind's story?

_____

_____

_____

It can be frustrating to see where you get stuck, but the very act of recognizing these patterns is essential to finding lasting pain relief and learning healthier ways to relate to the world. As the saying goes, "There are no mistakes in life, only lessons."

Yoga is very practical. Contrary to common misconceptions, yoga is not about trying to cultivate some "ideal" state in which we are always relaxed. Yoga is the skill of remaining aware and receptive to whatever arises in order to learn to be happier and healthier.

Also, are you at times connecting with simple being during your daily life? If not, take a moment right now to notice that, along with whatever else you're experiencing—seeing, hearing, thinking, feeling—at the center of these various experiences is a basic sense of your presence, what you call "I." Without this basic sense of yourself, none of these experiences could happen.

Take a few moments to clearly acknowledge this simple yet essential core of yourself. Like the stable axis around which a wheel revolves, simple being provides a reliable point of refuge you can return to and find your bearings.

WEEK 5

Riding the Waves of Pain

The mind settles as one cultivates friendliness, compassion, delight,
and equanimity toward all things, whether pleasant or painful, good or bad.
—Yoga Sutras of Patanjali (1:33)

Like all sensations, pain occurs in wavelike patterns. Some of these patterns, such as pain flares, may feel as if they will last forever—yet eventually they reach a peak and begin to subside. Other patterns may fluctuate quickly, such as a throbbing sensation in the knees after climbing stairs.

For many people, waves of pain are the most difficult to navigate. This is in part because pain is influenced by virtually everything in our lives, including our physical health, emotions, thoughts, relationships, and even past experiences (for additional details, see the "More About Pain" supplemental chapter available at http://www.newharbinger.com/43287).

Pain is also tricky because something that may be helpful in the short run may prove harmful if done too much. For example, bed rest for a sore back may be fine for one day, but lying in bed for a prolonged period brings on stiffness, deconditioning, and weight gain—resulting in increased pain and disability in the long run.

The harsh reality is that chronic pain is difficult to manage well because it is extremely complicated. The following two experiences highlight one aspect of this complexity: the fact that our emotions can affect our pain, both for better and worse.

Same Injury, Different Experience

Let's look at how the same injury to the same person can result in two different experiences:

A friend of ours was feeling quite anxious as she was running late to work on a snowy morning. In addition to having to drive very slowly and cautiously along the icy city roads, on that particular morning she had to drop off her daughter at school. In a hurry to get to her office, our friend slammed her thumb in the car door as she was getting out. Not surprising, her thumb throbbed for hours that day.

Several months later, this same friend was giddy with excitement as she drove to the airport to board a flight to Honolulu for a much-anticipated vacation. As she got out of her car, she slammed her thumb in the door. She hardly noticed any pain in her thumb that day; later she was surprised to notice that her thumb was bruised.

These two experiences highlight the fact that when you're excited and happy, you may hardly notice a potentially painful injury, but if you're anxious and worried, the same injury may hurt a lot more. This is not to say that your pain isn't real or is "all in your head." Because in fact, *the pain is always in your head*—but it's in your *neurology*, not your *psychology*. Remember, it's your brain that determines whether something is painful, and how you experience pain is influenced by a wide array of factors including what's going on for you physically, emotionally, mentally, and even spiritually.

How Pain Works

For centuries, pain was thought to function almost exclusively as a warning signal of physical injury. In the early 1600s, the French philosopher and scientist René Descartes studied human cadavers and theorized that, when a body part was injured, a signal traveled from the site of the injury to the brain, which would then command an appropriate action.

For example, if your finger was caught in a mouse trap, this would trigger an alarm signal from your finger to your brain, which would cause you to free your finger from the trap. This model assumed that specialized nerves, spread throughout the body, pick up pain signals and transmit them to the brain via the spinal cord. The signals were thought to travel just one way—from the injury to the brain. And the strength of the signals was thought to indicate the severity of injury, that is, stronger pain meant greater injury.

Many people, including some doctors, still think of pain in this way. Yet scientists began questioning this simplistic explanation in the mid-1900s because common battlefield situations during World War II defied this one-dimensional understanding of pain. For instance, military doctors noted that right after being seriously injured in combat, many soldiers felt little or no pain. This contradicted the way pain was thought to work. In contrast, soldiers who had a limb amputated nearly always continued to feel excruciating "phantom pain" that seemed to come from the limb that was no longer there—which makes no sense if pain is simply a signal transmitted from an injured body part.

Gate Control Model

To make sense of these unexpected situations, scientists developed a new theory for how pain works. First proposed in the mid-1960s, the gate control model hypothesized that there is a biochemical gateway located where nerves from various parts of the body connect to the spinal cord. When this gate is more fully open, pain signals pass more freely to the brain, so the person feels pain *more* intensely. When the gate closes substantially, signals can't pass as easily, so the person feels pain *less* intensely. Further, these scientists theorized that the opening and closing of this biochemical gate is influenced by a variety of factors, including a person's thoughts and emotions.

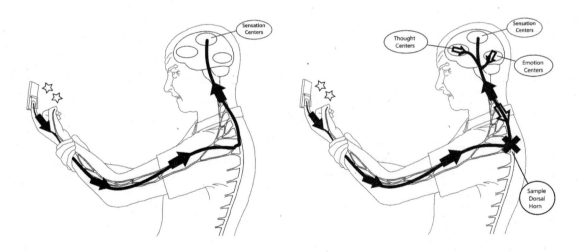

Pain Model Evolution: Single pathway to gate control

This model of pain has since been supported by thousands of studies. In fact, the gate control model has now been updated as the "neuromatrix model" (Melzack 1999). New research has revealed details not only about the "pain gate" in the spine but about the numerous influences within the brain itself that alter how pain signals are processed. For example, researchers discovered nerve pathways from the sensory, cognitive, and emotional centers in the brain down into the gate area (spinal dorsal horn), which helped solve the mystery of why a person may feel little pain from a major injury or experience ongoing pain from a missing limb.

Thoughts and emotions were found to strongly influence the perception of pain—with positive thoughts like joy and love "closing" the gate and thus dampening pain signals, and negative emotions like anger and fear "opening" the gate and thus heightening pain signals. In addition, scientists discovered that our bodies release lots of endorphins—the body's morphine-like natural painkillers—at times of severe injury, which usually closes down the pain gate (Butler and Moseley 2013). Endorphin release also increases during physical exercise, which explains the so-called "runner's high" when a marathoner may feel so much euphoria that they don't notice pain from blisters, bumps, or sprains.

How Mindful Yoga Can Help You Ride Waves of Pain

Pain's complexity may seem like bad news, since there is no simple solution for chronic pain. Most people who experience persistent pain find themselves—sooner or later—locked in a battle that absorbs a great deal of their attention, time, and energy. Sometimes it seems that the only alternative is to give up, to surrender everything, in an attempt to avoid more pain.

But there is also very good news related to pain's complexity, because many of the important influences on pain are at least partially under your control—and this means there is a much better alternative to constantly battling or giving up. Instead, *we invite you to explore changing your relationship to sensations, especially to the experience of painful and uncomfortable sensations. This is the essence of learning to ride the waves of pain,* and we've seen many people use this approach to relieve their pain and suffering.

Your skill in riding waves of various types—how you breathe, how you move (or don't move), how you direct you attention, how you deal with stress, how you think about and react emotionally to your situation and pain itself (your mind's story)—can change your relationship to sensations. This change powerfully affects not only the pain itself but also your overall quality of life.

Our Mindful Yoga studies have demonstrated improvements not just in pain but also in mood, fatigue, sleep, relaxation, invigoration, and healthy acceptance among people living with various types of persistent pain. Many people in these studies had been living with chronic pain for decades. And our studies have repeatedly demonstrated a "dose-response relationship"—that is, when people practiced Mindful Yoga strategies more, they experienced greater improvements.

Several essential elements of Mindful Yoga help promote a change in how you relate to pain. If you have been doing the recommended practices, you have already begun to shift your relationship to pain in the following five ways: breathing, postures, meditation, self-study, and keeping the company of truth.

Breathing

The Three-Part Breath practice affects your nervous system by triggering the relaxation response, which is the opposite of the fight-or-flight stress response, and involves a cascade of calming effects, such as slowing the heart rate. Relaxation feels pleasant, which is an emotional response that tends to close the pain gate. And it also facilitates widespread release of tense muscles throughout your body—and relaxed muscles don't ache like tight muscles.

This style of breathing also produces *invigoration,* which gives you more energy to do what you want to do—and that will indirectly affect your pain by reducing stress. Additional helpful breathing practices will be introduced in the coming weeks.

Postures

When movement hurts, people tend to stop moving—which can lead to a vicious cycle of inactivity. Without proper movement, the body gets stiff and out of shape, muscles become achy, and people often gain weight—which makes movement even more difficult and painful.

Mindful Yoga postures help you relearn a new way of moving—with self-compassion and awareness—taking movement to the point of challenge but avoiding strain. Practiced regularly, over time these gentle, healthy postures can enhance flexibility, strength, balance, endurance, and function—all of which can contribute to pain relief. These exercises also promote the release of pain-relieving endorphins (Tolahunase, Sagar, and Dada 2017; Yadav et al. 2012). Furthermore, these combined improvements allow people who have been struggling with pain to befriend their bodies again and to resume some of the activities they previously enjoyed.

Importantly, Mindful Yoga focuses on the *quality of your attention* as you move your body. When you apply mindful awareness to your posture practice, you gradually learn to free yourself from subtle patterns of reactivity, such as anxious thoughts, shallow breathing, and fear-related guarding patterns that prevent fluid movement—and all of these changes translate into less pain.

Moreover, as shown in our studies, the process of refining your relationship to your bodily sensations can gradually rewire your brain so that healthy movements that previously felt uncomfortable are no longer experienced as painful. This includes not just yoga postures but other daily life activities.

Meditation

During the meditation practice you learn to identify simple being and discover how to rest in this stable aspect of your experience. As you become more familiar with centering in this way, you find yourself calmer and you begin to recognize and feel a sense of love, of deep-down goodness, at your center—and these feelings help close the pain gate.

When your meditation practice progresses, as it did in Week 3 to include observing bodily sensations, you are further cultivating acceptance. Rather than struggling ineffectively to block out, resist, or otherwise escape your own experience, acceptance is working with what can be changed, such as the ways you pay attention to, think about, and emotionally react to pain. Studies have shown that acceptance of this sort leads to less pain, disability, emotional distress, and need of opioid medications (McCracken, Vowles, and Eccleston 2005; Vowles and McCracken 2008).

Self-Study and Keeping the Company of Truth

In Mindful Yoga, these two yoga tools are implemented primarily through informal practices woven into daily life—paying attention in the moment to riding the waves of breath, sensations, stress reactions, and the mind's stories—and by journaling in this workbook about what you are learning. Through this process of honest self-observation, you hopefully have noticed that your mind's narratives can often take you on unnecessary, unhelpful detours that heighten your stress level as well as your pain. If you persist in applying these wisdom teachings to your daily life, you will get better and better at riding all kinds of potentially stressful waves of experience.

Over the last few weeks, as you have practiced observing your mind's stories, you may have sometimes caught yourself immersed in *catastrophizing,* an unfortunately common habit of mind that involves imagining and ruminating on the worst possible outcomes. Examples of catastrophizing include: "This pain is so terrible that I may never recover" or "My spouse might leave me, and my children would suffer." Such thoughts are pain gate openers, and catastrophizing about pain is strongly associated with worsening of pain, poor response to medical treatment, increased anxiety and depression, and more disability (Keefe et al. 2004).

In addition, when people catastrophize, they lose confidence in their ability to cope. However, as shown in our Mindful Yoga for fibromyalgia study, when people learn to apply mindful awareness and cease to perpetuate these habits of mind, they report less tendency to catastrophize and significantly less pain (Carson et al. 2010; Carson et al. 2012).

Grace's Story

Grace had been a hairdresser, but once the first of her four children was born, she fully embraced being a stay-at-home mom and loved it. Her husband ran a construction company and provided the family with all the important necessities, including a lovely home by the river. Grace's life seemed idyllic until one morning, when her children were small, she was in a serious automobile accident. It took a couple of years, including two major spinal surgeries, for her to return to somewhat normal functioning—but by that time, she had been diagnosed with fibromyalgia.

Despite her determination not to allow the pain to take over, Grace began to do fewer of her favorite activities, including aerobic exercise. Frightened by the gradual worsening of pain, she also stopped taking her beloved walks by the river—and began neglecting some household chores.

As fear of worsening pain continued haunting her, Grace became depressed. She had always thought of herself as a cheerful person, but living with so much pain and fear took a toll on her. A friend suggested that a gentle yoga class might help, which led her to sign up for our Mindful Yoga course. At first she was unwilling to do the postures but liked the breathing and meditation practices. After hearing other students describe the benefits they were getting from the postures, Grace committed to doing at least a short posture practice each day.

During the fifth class, she shared that "for years I have tried to minimize taking my prescribed opioid meds, but usually I've needed them a few times a week. Now I've gone a whole month without taking them. It's such a great feeling to know that I am no longer dependent on opioids! If my pain increases now, I'm no longer afraid that it will just stay forever, I'm no longer terrified of hurting."

At the end of the eight-week course, Grace celebrated her oldest daughter's eighteenth birthday by taking her on a trip to Lake Tahoe. Later she recalled, "We had a great time. We were quite active, so I came home fairly sore. But unlike before, I didn't crash. I was able to make a 'soft landing' and resume my activities at home. The pain used to feel like a huge burden, but now I finally feel like I got my old self back again!"

Additional Tools for Riding the Waves of Pain

Here are some additional strategies that can help shift the way you relate to sensory experiences, including pain and related sensations, such as feeling distressed or fatigued. Keep in mind that generating this shift takes dedication and patience but ultimately results in less suffering and more joy and peace of mind.

Watching Sensations in a Nonreactive Way

This week, we will continue to refine our relationship to sensations. When you look closely, you can usually detect some variation in sensations. By learning to observe sensations in a curious, nonreactive way—that is, just noticing the sensations without getting involved in a mental story—you can often discover their dynamic qualities.

First, notice the *geography*—that is, the location of a strong sensation—and try to sense into its center. Next, sense into the periphery (outer edges) of the sensation. Notice what *qualities* are present. They might be vibrations, heat, tightness, sharpness, heaviness, tingling, or the like. Next, see whether the sensation stays exactly the same or *fluctuates*. Is there a change in intensity, quality, or location? Also, try to sense the *spaciousness* of the sensation, that is, the space that surrounds it. Notice what happens when you become more curious and inquisitive about sensations in these ways.

> Observe the dynamics of the sensation: geography, qualities, fluctuations, spaciousness.

Breathing into Sensation

Once you have explored the geography, quality, fluctuations, and spaciousness of sensations, next add "breathing into sensation," which can ease pain or discomfort. This practice involves directing your attention to those places that are hurting and inviting the life-giving energy of the breath into those areas. It is important to practice this skill with less difficult sensations first to make it easier to apply this skill when the pain gets strong.

When you engage in this practice, the air you breathe obviously does not pass beyond the lungs themselves. However, studies have demonstrated that when a person brings calm, focused attention to areas of their body, this is accompanied by increased blood flow and oxygen delivery to those areas, which can have healing effects (Lehrer et al. 1994; Violani and Lombardo 2003).

In addition, according to yogic texts, this practice of breathing into sensation directs vital energy, or *prana*, into the areas you focus on. Prana is described as the underlying life force that enlivens all living beings—similar to chi in traditional Chinese medicine—and is believed to convey significant healing effects.

Breathing into Sensation Practice

Begin by bringing curious and nonreactive attention to some area in your torso where there is *mild* discomfort. If possible, it might be helpful to place your hand there—for example, on your shoulder or chest. Practice directing your breath into this area. After welcoming a couple of breaths into this area, see what you notice about any changes in sensations in this area.

As a skill-building exercise, next try bringing breath into a specific area of your torso that has *little* or *no* discomfort. After "breathing" into the selected area for several moments, notice any effects of the practice.

It can also be very helpful to practice breathing into parts of the body where there is clearly no lung tissue. For example, bring attention into a hip and breathe into the hip for a couple of breaths. After a few moments, stay still and see what you notice in that hip.

Explore this practice for a few moments in different areas of the body and see what you discover.

How You Label Sensations

Words can have a powerful effect on how we perceive something. Each word is a seed that can grow into a story in the mind. For example, on a blustery winter day, if someone tells you, "The weather will be horrible," it's likely to affect you somewhat differently than if they say, "It's going to be cold and windy."

For many people, the word "pain" is strongly associated with negative experiences and prompts them to tense up and guard against anticipated suffering. This week, explore the effect of labeling by using the term "sensation" rather than "pain"—both in your internal dialogue and when talking with others. For example, rather than thoughts of "intense pain" you might label the experience as "intense sensation." If you practice nonjudgmental awareness of the sensations directly—and refine how you name the experience—you might notice a difference in how you feel. This practice of kind, curious self-inquiry often results in relief.

Reconnecting with Simple Being

Reconnecting with simple being can provide some refuge from pain. Resting into just being present offers a pause from the ongoing momentum of "mental time travel"—thoughts that race forward and backward in time, trying to avoid the pain you don't want and trying to get what you do want. Usually after a few moments of staying with simple being, the mind's thought waves calm down a bit, and that calm may also help you get clear about how best to go forward despite any tough sensations.

A Riptide of Pain

Occasionally a riptide of pain may threaten to pull you under. Although your instincts may be to fight by swimming against the current toward shore, that's the most dangerous thing you could do. Even elite swimmers can't swim out of riptides. Just as the safest way to navigate a riptide is to float or tread water until it has weakened and then swim diagonally out of the current, it's probably best to allow an overwhelming pain flare to wash through, rather than try to fight it with any particular strategy. Remember, all waves eventually do subside.

Week 5 Recommended Practice Schedule

Formal Practice

Record notes on the formal practice calendar. Jot down your practice times and observations on the weekly calendar provided at the end of this chapter.

Postures

Week 5 Yoga Posture Sequence. Turn to the "Mindful Yoga Posture Practices" section on page 133 and follow the instructions for Week 5; you can also follow along with the downloadable video available at http://www.newharbinger.com/43287. Practice every other day, at least three times this week. As you do the postures, continue to notice the mind's inner dialogue and commentary on the posture practice. Become aware of waves of discomfort that may arise—either as short waves or longer ones.

If a wave of pain moves through, notice what happens if you relabel it as a "sensation," and try exploring whether the sensation varies in intensity, quality, or location. See if you can sense the space surrounding the sensation. Finally, see if you can direct your breath toward that area and breathe into the sensation. Then resume your practice.

Breathing

Breathing into Sensation. Try to practice periodically every day while noticing whether this exercise impacts difficult sensations.

Meditation

Breath Through Sensing. Practice five times this week guided by the audio recording at http://www.newharbinger.com/43287. Again, the aim in meditation this week is to deepen your stability and flexibility of attention.

Informal Practice

Self-study. Throughout this week, become curious about the waves of pain sensations. Try out each of these ways of working with pain or discomfort at least once during the week:

- Watch sensations in a nonreactive way to see what you can discover about their locations, qualities, and dynamic or static nature.

- Breathe into sensation.

- Notice the effect of how you label the sensations. For example, if you label them as a "strong sensation" instead of "pain," see if that makes a difference.

- Reconnect with simple being. See if the mind's waves calm down a bit and whether you get clearer about how best to go forward despite the pain.

Keeping the company of truth. On the following worksheet, describe what you have observed and learned about the waves of pain.

Keeping the Company of Truth: Riding the Waves of Pain

Try out each of these ways of working with pain or discomfort at least once during the week: breathe watch sensations in a nonreactive way; breathe into sensation; notice the effect of how you label the sensations; reconnect with simple being.	Which of the four ways of riding waves of pain or discomfort did you use? Did that practice seem to make any difference? If so, briefly describe.
Day 1	
Day 2	
Day 3	
Day 4	
Day 5	
Day 6	
Day 7	

Week 5 Formal Practice—Riding the Waves of Pain

Please record time spent in each practice. Note any observations.

	Breath Breathing into Sensation	**Meditation** Breath Through Sensing	**Postures** Week 5	**Observations** What did you notice about waves of pain during your formal practice?
Day 1 Time				
Notes				
Day 2 Time				
Notes				
Day 3 Time				
Notes				

	Breath Breathing into Sensation	Meditation Breath Through Sensing	Postures Week 5	Observations What did you notice about waves of pain during your formal practice?
Day 4 Time				
Notes				
Day 5 Time				
Notes				
Day 6 Time				
Notes				
Day 7 Time				
Notes				

Week 5 Review

Before continuing, let's review what you have learned so far.

First, practice the Breath Through Sensing guided meditation at http://www.newharbinger .com/43287.

Next, briefly review your practice and observations from Week 5. Have you noticed any changes in how you experience strong sensations this week? Did you try—at least once— each of these strategies?

Yes   No

☐   ☐   Observing sensations in a kind and curious way, while exploring the geography, center and edges, qualities, fluctuations, and space around sensations.

☐   ☐   Breathing into sensation.

☐   ☐   Experimenting with using the label "strong sensation" instead of "pain."

☐   ☐   Resting into simple being.

Which seemed more effective for you this week? Please describe.

_____

_____

Did you use these strategies while doing the yoga postures, during meditation, or both?

_____

_____

Did you use these strategies during your daily life?

_____

_____

Describe how your formal and informal practices affected you.

_____

_____

_____

By now, you've had several weeks to discover what it's like to ride the waves of the mind's story. This can be a particularly challenging, yet rewarding, skill to develop. Once you're able to watch your mind's movements without being caught up in them, even for a minute, you may come to the clear realization that you don't have to believe everything your mind says! That insight usually brings a new sense of freedom.

It may be both a surprise and a relief to discover that you can have any kind of thought, but *you don't need to let any thought have you.* As you get better at riding the waves of your mind's stories, you will increasingly recognize that what these stories tell you, and what is actually happening at the moment, can be quite different. Knowing this allows you to avoid mulling over catastrophizing thoughts and to make better decisions about how to cope with pain and handle whatever challenges you may be facing.

Here are some common difficulties in observing the mind's stories, along with suggestions for addressing them:

I keep arguing with my mind.

When it becomes obvious that your mind is telling stories that are quite different from your direct experience—for example, "My pain never gets any better," when in fact your pain has calmed down a bit—you may feel tempted to get into an internal argument with your mind by asserting, "That's not true, right now it's better!"

This argument may also arise when the mind resists naming pain as a "tough sensation." But arguing with the mind is like jumping into quicksand: the more you use thoughts to try to counter other thoughts, the more stuck you become in a struggle with no end in sight.

The truth is, each and every thought is an idea *about* reality but is not the direct reality itself. Instead of buying into the frenzy of thoughts, try backing off and watching with curiosity; you will find that often thoughts settle on their own. Remember, your mind is really trying to help—it's just that it often jumps to conclusions as it loses track of what is actually happening, right now. Let this new relationship to the mind's stories be an experiment, not something you're forcing the mind to do.

A somewhat different challenge you may be having currently is the following:

I don't want to observe sensations.

For many people, observing and becoming curious about uncomfortable sensations seems counterintuitive: "Why should I choose to feel this pain?" is a common reaction. Begin the practice of exploring difficult sensations gently, for just two or three breaths. Just as you wouldn't try to cross the Mississippi before you could navigate a narrow stream, develop this skill gradually.

If you encounter considerable resistance to observing sensations, become curious about the resistance itself. Can you feel it in your body? What kinds of thoughts and emotions arise with the resistance? Let yourself get to know it. Remember, resistance is often an unconscious habit and can quickly elevate pain. Refining how you relate to painful sensations includes refining your relationship with resistance as well.

WEEK 6

Riding the Waves of Emotions

All emotions are rooted in love... So even those feelings that end up causing us suffering actually spring from a kernel of love.

—Joel Morwood, contemporary meditation teacher

Our words reflect the reality that we experience emotions *physically*, often in particular parts of our bodies. Phrases such as "gut feelings" and "heartfelt" are prime examples of the strong link between how we feel and where we experience these feelings. The heart, in particular, is often the center of sensations that convey our emotional states. Bad news can make our "heart sink" while good new might make our "heart rejoice."

Like all energies, our emotions move in a wavelike pattern: arising, peaking, and eventually subsiding. Some of these waves of the heart can throw almost all human beings off balance at various times, particularly those involving difficult emotions such as anxiety, sadness, anger, frustration, or fear. Typically, such feelings are accompanied by troublesome thought patterns that often act like gasoline poured on a fire, fueling these unsettling emotions. For example, someone who felt their heart sink when they lost their job may spin this understandable feeling of disappointment into disastrous despair, with thoughts such as, "I'm a failure," "I'll never get a decent job," "I'll wind up alone and homeless." If this person is living with chronic pain, these catastrophizing thoughts would escalate their pain.

Naturally, when we're feeling uncomfortable sensations, there is most often an emotional response to this experience. These waves of emotions can be fueled by thoughts such as, "It's only going to get worse!" Before long, such thoughts become linked with the simultaneous experiences of emotional upset and pain via the "neurons that fire together, wire together" conditioning pattern that governs *neuroplasticity*. This linking of our thought patterns with our emotional reactions and pain means that when a similar thought arises in the future, there is a tendency for it to activate similar emotional and pain reactions.

It's like clicker-training a puppy to sit. The puppy first learns to sit by pairing the command "sit" with a tasty treat. Then the sound of the clicker is also paired with "sit" and a treat. Through this pairing, the pup's brain learns that the clicker indicates a treat is coming. Eventually, the sound of the clicker and sitting become wired together, such that the clicker alone triggers the puppy to sit, without the need for a treat.

With regard to pain, fortunately, the neural linking of thought patterns with uncomfortable sensations is a soft-wired process, meaning that it's reversible, assuming the person learns to refrain from jumping into catastrophizing waves of thought. In contrast, however, research shows that the parts of the brain involved in processing difficult emotions such as anxiety, fear, and sadness physically overlap to a great extent with areas that process chronic pain (Vachon-Presseau et al. 2016). In other words, *physical pain and emotional pain naturally co-occur.*

How Mindful Yoga Can Help You Ride Waves of Emotions

Yoga can help you cope with difficult emotions—and how your emotions affect your pain—in a variety of ways. Cultivating mindful awareness, both in movement and stillness practices, has been shown to improve mood (Carlson and Garland 2005; Carson et al. 2004; Holzel et al. 2011). In our Mindful Yoga studies, improvements in mood have coincided with improvements in pain as well (Carson et al. 2010; Carson et al. 2016; Carson et al. 2012; Carson et al. 2009; Carson et al. 2007).

One reason for these mood improvements is because yoga postures promote the release of endorphins (the body's natural opioids) and also induce a bodily relaxation response that brings about a positive shift in mood (Streeter et al. 2010; Yadav et al. 2012). Yoga breathing exercises can also produce a powerful relaxation response that almost immediately triggers a noticeable positive change in mood and also in pain (Martin et al. 2012). Importantly, your breath is the only physiologic function that is under both voluntary and involuntary control—that is, you can intentionally redirect your breath pattern or allow your body to automatically continue to breathe.

When you consciously regulate your breath, it provides a unique doorway into your mind-body connection. This powerful interactive relationship between breath, mind, and body has long been recognized by yoga masters, including Patanjali, who nearly two thousand years ago wrote, "Physical illness and related problems are accompanied by emotional distress and despair, trembling, and disturbed breathing. But by regulating the breath, especially by lengthening the exhalation, calm is restored" (Carson and Carson 2018). And this calm involves not only calmer breathing but also calmer emotions and calmer sensations, especially sensations that feel painful.

Extended Exhalation

Specific breathing techniques, such as the Extended Exhalation practice that follows, are designed to produce wide-ranging effects. Extended Exhalation involves gradually increasing your exhalation until it is longer than your inhalation. Even an exhalation that is only slightly longer than the inhalation can induce a calming effect, because it causes the vagus nerve (which runs from the neck down through the diaphragm) to signal to your brain to turn on the relaxation response (Berzin 2019).

The Extended Exhalation practice also decreases anxiety, including anxiety about pain, by helping to clear carbon dioxide from the blood stream. A common response to pain—or fear of pain—is breath holding, something you may not even be aware that you're doing. But when you hold your breath or breathe shallowly, it creates a buildup of carbon dioxide, which leads to an increase of anxiety reactions in the nervous system. Tools such as Three-Part Breath and Extended Exhalation help keep carbon dioxide from building up and can bring a greater sense of ease to the system (Busch et al. 2012).

Extended Exhalation Practice

This breathing practice is not meant to be your natural ongoing breath. It should be used periodically, when the body or mind feels stressed. Always stop if you feel any lightheadedness or dizziness, and then rest in the natural flow of breath.

To begin, sit or recline in a comfortable position. Close your eyes and turn your attention to your breath. Breathe in and out through your nose.

Place one palm on your abdomen and take a few relaxed breaths, feeling the abdomen expand on the inhalation and gently sink on the exhalation. With your palm on your abdomen, mentally count the length of each inhalation and exhalation for several more breaths.

Once you have a sense of the length of the in-breath and out-breath, begin to balance the breath. To do this, invite the inhalation and the exhalation to be about the same length. Spend a few breaths finding this balance—but please avoid any

---

struggle or strain. Just do your best to make your in-breath about as long as your out-breath.

As the inhalation and exhalation equalize, gradually increase the length of your exhalation by one count by gently contracting the abdomen as you exhale. Stay with this pattern—the exhalation one count longer than the inhalation—for a few breaths. Then, as long as the breath feels smooth and relaxed, and there is no sense of dizziness, explore lengthening the exhalation by another count of one. For example, if your breath ratio is 4 counts in to 5 counts out, see what it feels like to try a ratio of 4 counts in to 6 counts out. Again, make sure there is no experience of strain as the exhalation increases. Explore this breath rhythm for a few moments.

Riding the Wave of Emotions

Mindful Yoga practices can also serve as a laboratory for intentionally working with difficult emotions so that they cease to fuel the persistence of chronic pain. In yoga postures, you are invited to assume challenging positions and then notice responses of the physical body, the emotional heart, and the thinking mind. This practice cultivates greater awareness of how the body and the mind react to challenges. It also enhances your ability to observe mental narratives without fusing with these thoughts or being overwhelmed by the sensations. This process begins to shift you away from unconsciously "rehearsing" mental narratives that accentuate pain.

Similarly, learning to observe the reactions of the emotional heart without fueling such reactions with the mind's stories is also an important tool for working skillfully with pain. Often when an emotional current arises in response to pain or other stressful experiences, there is a subtle—or sometimes more obvious—thought that is either driving or perpetuating the emotional current. For example, recalling a heated conversation with a neighbor not only stirs the memory of the encounter but also how you felt, or the emotional tenor, during that argument.

It is almost impossible to attend to thinking and feeling at the same time.

Generally, our mental habit is to continue retelling stories—either to ourselves or to someone we know—about how they were wrong, why we were right, and so forth. Regardless of the accuracy of these stories, they end up stimulating our emotional waves—making our emotional experience stronger or making it last longer. Learning to steady attention on the bare emotion, without adding fuel from the story, is an invaluable skill. This allows the waves of emotions to move through your system so that they can subside and not amplify your pain.

Interestingly, it is almost impossible to attend to thinking and feeling at the same time. By focusing attention on the pure experience of really sensing—fully feeling an emotion—rather than thinking about what stirred it or how to make things different, you allow the wave of emotion to peak and then diminish. In contrast, when you feed the spinning wheel of the mind with your attention, it energizes the emotional waves and can ramp up pain.

It's important to recognize that human emotions are complex, essential components of who we are. Sometimes emotions can be distressing, and it's common to try to push them away. For example, you might be embarrassed by feeling angry at a loved one, which might cause you to attempt to repress—or block—this feeling. The result can be an inner struggle that eventually leads to further problems, including creating distance in your relationships. Holding on to anger or other difficult emotions, rather than skillfully letting them move through your system, only worsens pain.

Rather than avoiding distressing emotions, a different approach can be helpful, even though it may seem counterintuitive at first glance: learning to simply feel the various emotions as they arise, peak, and subside—much like you have been learning to observe the wavelike patterns of physical sensations.

We can think of emotions as the soundtrack of our lives: without various moods and emotions, our lives would become quite dry, monotonous, and meaningless. In fact, when most people go to the movies or read novels, they seek out plots that are quite dramatic, so that they can temporarily—but less personally—experience powerful emotions of fear, love, sadness, joy, and the like.

Rather than block emotions, we can learn to welcome each one and discover what it conveys about life. This capacity to recognize, remain open to, and effectively cope with various emotions is the skill of riding the waves of emotions. In research terms, this ability is known as *emotional intelligence,* and evidence shows that the more "emotionally intelligent" a person is, the less likely they are to suffer from either temporary or chronic pain (Baker et al. 2016; Doherty et al. 2017).

This week, we invite you to be willing to temporarily explore your various emotions. You will discover how each different emotion—such as joy, sorrow, contentment, anger, fear, and love—makes itself known via distinctive sensory qualities. This will feel similar to the practice introduced in Week 5 of becoming curious about the sensory geography, qualities, and wavelike patterns of pain.

Emotion Laboratory

Consider the emotion of joy. To practice this, briefly generate a sense of joy by recalling a moment when you felt joyful. Let the memory become vivid, remembering where you were, what happened, who was there. As the feeling of joy comes into focus, however mild or strong, turn your attention from the *memory* of joy to the *feeling* of joy. Notice where you feel the emotion of joy in your body.

Many people describe feeling joy in their heart region, but others feel it elsewhere, such as in their face. Where do you feel it? What are the qualities you notice about joy? For example, does it feel light or heavy? Warm or cool (or neither)? Does it seem to vibrate or does it feel solid? Does it seem to expand or contract? See if you can stay with sensing the *feeling of* joy rather than becoming involved in thoughts about the feeling.

Next, invite forth the feeling of sorrow by recalling a time when you lost something or someone you cared about. Don't worry, you won't have to feel this for long, and the process of opening to sorrow will boost your emotional flexibility. Once you can sense some degree of sorrow, shift your attention from the memory to the feeling and again inquire: Where do I feel this emotion in my body? What are the particular qualities I notice when sorrow is present: light or heavy, warm or cool, stationary or flowing?

Now try this same process with four other emotions: contentment, anger, fear, and love. Where do you feel each emotion? What are the sensory qualities each emotion elicits? The more you practice getting to know the essential nature of your emotions, *without* habitually blocking or fueling them, you build emotional intelligence. You will be able to stay present as emotions arise, allowing the waves to move through without holding their energy in place, which otherwise would only tax the system and further fuel chronic pain.

An audio recoding of the Emotion Laboratory Exercise is available at http://www.newharbinger.com/43287.

Surviving an Emotional Tsunami

Sometimes the waves of emotions we feel are akin to emotional tsunamis, so persistent or strong that any effort to calm them only makes things worse. In these cases, it's best to let such tsunamis wash over and through you, knowing that the intensity will eventually peak and then begin to settle on its own. Again, two primary yogic principles—acceptance and love—are essential to navigating through intense emotional turbulence:

Acceptance can lessen the suffering that comes from struggling and denying, which may seem to work in the short run but backfires in the long run, leading to even stronger emotions and ultimately more pain. Yoga philosophy teaches that "You yourself can be your own best friend or worst enemy."

Love invites you to be patient and kind with yourself as well as with others. Remember, all waves eventually do subside. Love of some kind, in fact, is actually at the root of all emotions, and all emotions can be traced back to love. For example, fear arises from anticipated loss of someone, something, or an idea we love. Likewise, sadness reflects having lost someone, something, or an idea we love; anger arises when someone, something, or an idea we love has been harmed.

When we can recognize and trace a difficult emotion to its root in what we love, then even though that emotion doesn't disappear, its effect shifts as the feeling of love is simultaneously aroused. And honoring the love underlying various emotions can be a valuable tool for not only learning to ride emotional waves but also for calming pain, because love is a pain gate closer—it dampens the intensity of uncomfortable sensations.

Another way to evoke the healing presence of love is to do the audio-guided Meditation on Deep-Down Goodness, which can be found at http://www.newharbinger.com/43287.

Annie's Story

Annie was an elementary-school teacher who specialized in working with kids with special needs. At age forty-five, she found out that she had metastatic breast cancer—a shocking diagnosis that changed everything for Annie, her husband, and their two young children. All of the family rhythms were impacted by Annie's medical appointments and treatments, after which she always felt very fatigued and sometimes excruciating pain. Although Annie had ample professional skills and experience for dealing with stressful classroom situations, facing this life-threatening illness felt devastating.

Annie enrolled in our Mindful Yoga course because she wanted tools to relax out of her almost perpetual state of panic. The gentle poses felt nourishing to her body and helped her begin to reconnect with a sense of well-being. But she shared that, although she loved the sense of ease she experienced during the class, it wasn't long before the real and overwhelming experience of cancer would again agitate her system.

One day, during her home meditation practice, Annie noticed a familiar but subtle thought: "Good parents aren't sick. I can't parent while going through treatment." She began to recognize how this thought was influencing how she interacted with her family, how it was driving her to withdraw from her children and husband. By applying the skill she'd learned in yoga of observing her mind's stories in a nonreactive way, Annie was able to trace her persistent anxiety to its source, which was the deep love she felt for her family. She began to apply this insight over and over—each time she found herself becoming highly anxious, she turned her attention to feeling how much she cared for her husband and children. As she did so, she often noticed that the pain diminished.

Annie said this realization helped her feel empowered to honor how her body was struggling and yet be as present as possible with those she loved. It helped her recognize that although she may be hurting, feeling ill, or fatigued, she could still listen to her children's stories about their day, could still sit at the dinner table, could still cuddle with her husband. For Annie, the combination of the relaxing and nourishing dimension of the postures, the clarity that came with the meditation, and the ability to trace her upsetting feelings to their source in the relationships she most loved, helped her find peace, hope, and pain relief amid the challenges of her cancer journey.

Week 6 Recommended Practice Schedule

Formal Practice

Record notes on the formal practice calendar. Jot down your practice times and observations on the weekly calendar provided at the end of this chapter.

Postures

Week 6 Yoga Posture Sequence. Turn to the "Mindful Yoga Posture Practices" section on page 133 and follow the instructions for Week 6; you can also follow along with the downloadable video available at http://www.newharbinger.com/43287. Practice every other day, at least three times this week. As you do the postures, continue to notice your mind's inner dialogue and commentary on the posture practice. Become aware of waves of emotion that may arise either as short waves or longer ones. If you notice any waves of emotion, see if you can pause to notice the location and qualities of the feelings, and extend kindness to this aspect of yourself.

Breathing

Extended Exhalation. Try to practice periodically (at least once or twice) each day while noticing whether this breath practice impacts the waves of emotions.

Meditation

Breath Through Thoughts. Now that you have had several weeks of informally observing your mind weave stories about various daily activities—and also noticing the mind's inner dialogue while doing yoga posture exercises—it's time to deepen this aspect of your practice. Go to http://www.newharbinger.com/43287 to access the audio-guided Breath Through Thoughts meditation. For many people, refining the skill of observing the mind's activities without getting constantly lost in thought is enormously helpful for avoiding all kinds of pitfalls that can make pain and other problems worse. So your meditation practice this week will be extended to include both 1) watching your mind's internal flow of commentary and images, and also 2) noticing waves of emotions as they make themselves known. Practice at least five times this week, guided by the audio recording.

Informal Practice

Self-study. Become curious about the emotions that naturally arise in your day-to-day experience. See if you can just sense the *feeling* of the emotion rather than focusing on the *thought* or story that is fueling the emotion. Try out each of these ways of working with upsetting emotions at least once during the week:

- Practice Emotion Laboratory.

- Practice Extended Exhalation.

- Trace upsetting feelings to their source in something you love.

- Do the Meditation on Deep-Down Goodness, which can be found at http://www.newharbinger.com/43287.

Keeping the company of truth. On the following worksheet, describe what you have observed and learned about working with various emotions.

Keeping the Company of Truth: Riding the Waves of Emotions

Try out each of these ways of working with upsetting emotions at least once during the week: practice Emotion Lab; practice Extended Exhalation; trace upsetting feelings to their source in something you love; and do the Meditation on Deep-Down Goodness.	Which of the four ways of riding emotions did you use? Did that practice seem to make any difference? If so, briefly describe.
Day 1	
Day 2	
Day 3	
Day 4	
Day 5	
Day 6	
Day 7	

Week 6 Formal Practice—Riding the Waves of Emotion

Please record time spent in each practice. Note any observations.

	Breath Extended Exhalation	**Meditation** Breath Through Thoughts	**Postures** Week 6	**Observations** What did you notice about any waves of emotion during your formal practice?
Day 1 Time				
Notes				
Day 2 Time				
Notes				
Day 3 Time				
Notes				

	Breath Extended Exhalation	Meditation Breath Through Thoughts	Postures Week 6	Observations What did you notice about any waves of emotion during your formal practice?
Day 4 Time				
Notes				
Day 5 Time				
Notes				
Day 6 Time				
Notes				
Day 7 Time				
Notes				

Week 6 Review

Before proceeding further, let's review what you have learned so far.

First, practice the audio-guided Breath Through Thoughts meditation at http://www.newharbinger.com/43287.

Next, review Week 6 and answer the following questions:

What was it like to ride the waves of emotional ups and downs?

_____

_____

Did you try the Emotion Laboratory, Extended Exhalation, tracing upsetting emotions back to the love that underlies them, and the Meditation on Deep-Down Goodness?

_____

_____

Were you able to use any of these skills during posture or meditation practice? Did you use them during your daily activities?

_____

_____

Describe how your formal and informal practices affected you.

_____

_____

_____

During the previous week, your recommended meditation practice had been extended to noticing emotional currents and observing thoughts.

I'm simply lost in thoughts throughout meditation.

Learning to observe thoughts coming and going without fusing with them is considered an advanced form of meditation. As you've meditated this past week, you've probably noticed a pattern that is sometimes called "monkey mind": your attention keeps jumping from one topic or concern to another in what may seem an endless cycle, and you often feel lost in the mix. Don't be discouraged!

Like any skill, it takes a good bit of patient practice before you are able to stay afloat and surf the waves of your mind without fusing with your thoughts and ending up confused. Persist in your practice but in a relaxed and compassionate way—not trying too hard, yet not becoming lax.

Taking Stock

As you near the end of this journey, here are some key questions:

Have you developed, at least to some extent, a daily yoga practice? Which practices are you able to include most days: breathing, postures, meditation, informal strategies? Which ones have you not incorporated?

_____

_____

Why are you drawn to the practices you've been doing most often? Are they easier? Are they less time demanding? Are they more rewarding? In what ways are they helping you?

_____

_____

What barriers are keeping you from including the practices you haven't done? Do they seem harder? Is there something about them you're avoiding or resisting?

_____

_____

Importantly, are you noticing any changes in how you feel day to day? For example, is your pain somewhat better? How about your mood? What are you noticing about your outlook as you engage in your daily activities? Are you having insights into how your mind works? Are you more often aware of the choices you make and less often running on autopilot?

Describe what you have discovered regarding insights you've had into how to better navigate life's challenges. List any changes you've noticed.

_____

_____

_____

_____

_____

_____

_____

_____

_____

_____

_____

Is there something more you hoped to get out of this program that hasn't yet come your way? If so, what were you hoping for? In our work helping people with chronic pain, it's clear that *changes only come with practice.* If you'd like to get more out of this program, please consider redoubling your efforts during the last two weeks so that *you practice every day— even for just ten or fifteen minutes—*to see if that will make a difference.

WEEK 7

Riding the Waves of Fatigue

All the worlds may be given to you, but if you will not be allowed to sleep,
you would rather say, "Let me sleep. I do not want any world."

—Swami Krishnananda

Chronic pain can be exhausting. Many people with chronic pain say that fatigue is their most distressing symptom. While everyone feels tired occasionally, chronic pain sufferers often report feeling tired *all the time.* This is partly because when pain is present, your central nervous system is working overtime to attempt to figure out and adapt to the pain. And when you're tired, every task, every activity, can feel like a burden. When that's the case, many people become chronically worried about getting things done—and worrying just adds to the exhaustion.

A major problem that compounds fatigue is poor sleep. Sound sleep is crucial for our physical and mental health. Inadequate sleep increases the risk of accidents and poor performance, and the resulting lack of energy can interfere with many daily activities, negatively affecting memory and mood.

Not surprising, people who don't sleep well are at greater risk of developing a chronic pain condition. Emerging neuroscience shows a complex interrelationship between pain and sleep, with poor sleep exacerbating pain sensitivity, and pain adversely affecting sleep quality. A key finding is that poor sleep impairs the brain's mechanisms for modulating pain signals, making a person more vulnerable to developing widespread, persistent pain (Finan, Goodin, and Smith 2013).

For example, women with fibromyalgia typically have little slow-wave sleep—which is the deeper, restorative stage of sleep—and also may experience a kind of disturbance called an "alpha intrusion," which means that they wake up (or come close to waking up) several times a night. Both of these concerns—lack of slow-wave sleep and intrusions of wakeful-ness—are related to chronic muscle soreness and fatigue (Van Houdenhove and Egle 2004). Studies also indicate that when people with rheumatoid arthritis experience sleep depriva-tion, the number of joints that are painful and overall pain severity becomes elevated (Irwin et al. 2012).

Like all natural phenomenon, fatigue follows a wavelike pattern—building, peaking, and subsiding. These waves can occur on a daily basis—for example, waking up tired, then feeling better after breakfast, with fatigue gradually building throughout the day to a peak in the late afternoon. And fatigue can also occur in longer, weekly wave patterns—for example, feeling very tired during a portion of the week and less tired on the weekend.

Breaking the Fatigue Cycle

When you're exhausted, moving your body may be the last thing you feel like doing. But surprisingly, there is strong evidence that low-intensity exercise can actually help boost energy and relieve fatigue. Particularly for people who are sedentary and fatigued, gentle movement—such as doing yoga postures or going for a short walk—may be better than a nap for combatting tiredness (O'Connor and Puetz 2005; Puetz, Flowers, and O'Connor 2008). Making regular physical activity a habit is associated with increased feelings of energy and decreased feelings of fatigue (Puetz, O'Connor, and Dishman 2006).

More specific, research confirms that yoga postures are effective for boosting energy levels and maintaining fitness (Wood 1993). Mindful Yoga includes the benefits of gentle

> **When cancer patients spent more time practicing yoga, their fatigue was lower the next day.**

movement in combination with many other helpful mental and emotional tools, which together have been shown to be particu-larly effective in breaking the fatigue cycle. Our fibromyalgia and breast cancer studies showed improvements in fatigue and sleep disturbance, and our metastatic breast cancer study found a par-ticularly lasting connection between Mindful Yoga practice and reduced fatigue. When women spent more time practicing yoga, their fatigue was lower the next day.

Acceptance Means Less Struggle

By now you've had some practice with acceptance—being willing to acknowledge the experience you're already having, rather than wasting precious energy on wishing that things were somehow different. In dealing with fatigue, acceptance means acknowledging that some aspects of fatigue can't be changed. The well-known prayer wisely recommends making peace with this reality and having "the serenity to accept the things I cannot change."

But accepting fatigue doesn't mean crawling into bed and pulling the covers up over your head! Sometimes it may be skillful to take a short nap when you're tired. And it's important to practice good sleep habits: setting a regular bedtime, establishing a relaxing sleep-time routine, not having caffeine after 2 p.m., and avoiding staring at computer and phone screens within two hours before going to sleep.

Accepting the reality of fatigue can also mean recognizing when you are most vulnerable to feeling tired, learning how to pace yourself, and scheduling activities wisely. For example, if you tend to feel tired when you wake up and need time to "get your motor running," avoid scheduling early classes or appointments.

Love Means Doing What Helps

Love is also essential in helping you ride the waves of fatigue. Here, love translates into taking good care of yourself, with the understanding that "charity begins at home." For example, when your flight is preparing to take off, you are reminded to secure your own oxygen mask before helping others. Providing necessary self-care is sometimes misunderstood as selfishness, but it's important to recognize that you can only help others if you have a measure of strength and wisdom yourself.

Especially when you are tired, it's important not to force issues—whether they are practical matters or emotional concerns—as this tendency can cause more harm than good and contribute to more fatigue.

It's also critical to take breaks as needed and to avoid pushing yourself. It's not uncommon for people dealing with chronic pain to experience good days and bad, and to have a tendency to push themselves to accomplish everything on their to-do list on a day when they feel good. All too often, this results in an escalation of exhaustion and pain, sometimes to the point of being unable to get out of bed.

To more skillfully ride the waves of fatigue, practice activity pacing—do a little, then rest a little. We model this skill on the yoga mat by doing a posture, then resting and noticing what's present. Our hope is that you can take this skill off the yoga mat and into your daily life—for example, after you perform an activity, take a break.

Activity pacing also involves not packing an unreasonable amount of activities into your day. And if you must perform a particularly demanding activity, schedule it at your peak energy time, then plan for a period of rest and recovery afterward.

When you're moving through Mindful Yoga postures, maintain a sense of stability and comfort in each pose, which involves finding the appropriate balance between effort and relaxation, courage and caution, doing and undoing. See if you can embrace this same balanced mindset as you go through your daily activities.

For example, if you're driving in heavy traffic, do your best to stay alert yet relaxed—perhaps by softening the grip of your hands on the steering wheel, keeping your breath flowing comfortably, and releasing any tension in your shoulders. Only use the energy you need for the task. If you're working around the house or yard, can you stay connected to how you feel physically and emotionally, and back off if you feel yourself overdoing it?

If the mind's story gets hyperfocused on fatigue—such as "I'm so tired that I just can't get anything finished. I feel worthless!"—don't let these thoughts get the best of you. The simple facts may be that 1) you often feel tired, and 2) fatigue is more common when a person has chronic pain. So adjustments are certainly called for, as with any major challenge in life. Recognize that being tired is a part of being human and that fatigue comes in waves. With practice and patience, you can skillfully learn how to cultivate energy and make the best use of your physical, emotional, and mental resources. Rather than beat yourself up for the human tendency to get tired, try kind self-understanding instead.

Yogic Sleep

Most of us are used to being either alert or relaxed, but not both at once. Being *both deeply relaxed and fully alert at the same time* is at the heart of a simple yet powerful meditation practice called *yoga nidra* ("yogic sleep"). Rooted in ancient teachings that focus on simple being and understanding the true nature of awareness, yoga nidra can reveal "an unshakable equilibrium that is present under all circumstances and situations," writes psychologist and yoga therapist Richard Miller. Research suggests that this practice can relieve stress, enhance sleep, reduce pain, and boost resilience in groups ranging from veterans with PTSD to college students (Eastman-Mueller et al. 2013; Miller 2003; Stankovic 2011).

The relaxation practice that you learned in the earlier weeks of this book is a sort of mini yoga nidra. The full yoga nidra practice goes even deeper. If you've ever experienced a moment of insight in that transitional period when you're just waking up or just about to fall asleep, you may be aware of the potential to connect with your deeper inner resources. Yoga nidra develops and enhances this connection with your inborn intelligence and bring its lessons into your daily life. We offer our yoga nidra guided meditation at http://www.newhar binger.com/43287.

George's Story

A soft-spoken man with distinguished white hair, George was about to retire after a satisfying career in education when he began experiencing a variety of unusual symptoms. He found himself walking with short, shuffling steps, his handwriting got smaller, and he became severely constipated. His doctor diagnosed him with Parkinson's disease, and as it progressed during the next few years, he developed chronic pain related to the unremitting muscle tension that is common in people with this disorder. George also struggled with profound fatigue, another characteristic of Parkinson's.

After trying many approaches to relieve his pain and fatigue, George enrolled in our Mindful Yoga program on the advice of his physician. During the first several weeks, he did his best to keep up but often became frustrated by his unreliable balance and tremors that made the practices very challenging.

When he was introduced to yoga nidra, however, George was surprised to find that his tremors settled, and he was able to stay much more focused during this practice. After yoga nidra ended, George found that his pain was almost undetectable for the first time in years. He also felt more energized than he had in a long time. This gave him hope that he had very helpful tools to continue to navigate the journey of Parkinson's disease.

Week 7 Recommended Practice Schedule

Formal Practice

Record notes on the formal practice calendar. Jot down your practice times and observations on the weekly calendar provided at the end of this chapter.

Postures

Week 7 Yoga Posture Sequence. Turn to the "Mindful Yoga Posture Practices" section on page 133 and follow the instructions for Week 7; you can also follow along with the downloadable video available at http://www.newharbinger.com/43287. Practice every other day, at least three times this week. As you do the postures, continue to notice the mind's inner dialogue and commentary on the posture practice. Become aware of waves of fatigue that may arise either as short waves or longer waves. If you feel a wave of fatigue, see if you can pause and rest for a few breaths and then resume the practice.

Breathing

Three-Part Breath. Practice periodically each day (at least once or twice) while noticing whether this impacts fatigue.

Meditation

Breathe Through Thoughts. Practice at least four times this week, guided by the audio recording available at http://www.newharbinger.com/43287. This week will focus on deepening your stability and flexibility of attention.

Yoga Nidra. This practice guides you gradually through a process of deep bodily relaxation, while remaining awake and aware of simple being. Go to http://www.newharbinger.com/43287 to access the audio-guided Yoga Nidra meditation. Some people fall asleep as they initially explore this practice. However, if you sleep too long, or too close to bedtime, you may have a hard time getting to sleep at night. So if possible, practice yoga nidra earlier rather than later in the day. Alternatively, you can explore using yoga nidra to help you to sleep better at night. In that case, practice yoga nidra just before bedtime and then go ahead and tuck yourself in. Practice at least three times this week.

Informal Practice

Self-study. Become curious about waves of fatigue. Practice being kind with yourself when fatigue gets overwhelming. Reconnect with simple being, just noticing you are present, even in the midst of fatigue.

Keeping the company of truth. On the following worksheet, describe what you have observed and learned about fatigue. How do your body, emotions, and thoughts respond to these waves?

Keeping the Company of Truth: Riding the Waves of Fatigue

If you feel fatigued today, try doing yoga postures and/or yoga nidra to help you ride the waves of fatigue.	Did doing yoga postures and/or yoga nidra help you ride the waves of fatigue? If so, briefly describe.
Day 1	
Day 2	
Day 3	
Day 4	
Day 5	
Day 6	
Day 7	

Week 7 Formal Practice—Riding the Waves of Fatigue

Record time spent in each practice. Note any observations.

	Meditation Yoga Nidra	Meditation Breath Through Thoughts	Postures Week 7	Observations What did you notice about waves of fatigue during your formal practice?
Day 1 Time				
Notes				
Day 2 Time				
Notes				
Day 3 Time				
Notes				

	Meditation Yoga Nidra	Meditation Breath Through Thoughts	Postures Week 7	Observations What did you notice about waves of fatigue during your formal practice?
Day 4 Time				
Notes				
Day 5 Time				
Notes				
Day 6 Time				
Notes				
Day 7 Time				
Notes				

Week 7 Review

Before going further, let's review what you have learned so far.

First, practice the Breathe Through Thoughts guided meditation.

Next, briefly review your practice and observations from Week 7.

Were you able to notice variations in the waves of fatigue?

_____

_____

What were the responses to the waves of fatigue: body, emotional heart, and thinking mind?

_____

_____

Were you able to extend kindness toward yourself when the waves of fatigue were strong?

_____

_____

What was the experience of yoga nidra like? How did it impact the waves of fatigue or any of the other waves of experience?

_____

_____

Could you rest into simple being, even during the big waves of fatigue?

_____

_____

Describe how your formal and informal practices affected you.

_____

_____

_____

As you start Week 8 here are some key questions to consider:

- Can you commit to practicing more often during this last week of the program?

- What would it be like to explore the practices that are less appealing? There may be a hidden treasure waiting to be discovered.

Continuing the Journey to Pain Relief

Rising, water's still water, falling back, it is water,
will you give me a hint how to tell them apart?
Because someone has made up the word "wave,"
do I have to distinguish it from water?

—Kabir (fifteenth-century Indian poet)

Congratulations on making it to the final week of the eight-week Mindful Yoga program! After spending decades helping people who live with chronic pain, we know how difficult persistent pain can be. So please applaud yourself for the time and effort you've put into applying the wisdom of the yoga tradition to your life.

Although the structured part of this program is ending, your personal journey, of course, continues. In this final chapter, we'll briefly review what you have learned and help you design your own practice to serve you for the rest of your life. Whatever helpful insights and skills you have gained through this book, this is just the beginning.

If you continue to practice yoga regularly, not only will your pain get better, your entire life will be gradually transformed in deep and rewarding ways—as was the case for Paula, a prime example of how a yoga practice can help you find ease in body and mind.

Paula's Story

A retired insurance salesperson in her late sixties, Paula had suffered from low-back pain for most of her adult life. She also experienced persistent pain in her arms and shoulders after having a mastectomy and radiation for breast cancer when she was in her mid-fifties.

Determined to "get things done," Paula tried to ignore and override her pain—pushing herself excessively to clean, garden, and do other activities. As a result, her pain would flare up and she would "crash," feeling as if she had to crawl into bed and stop moving. When this happened, her thoughts became dominated by memories of past struggles—including her divorce and losing her last job. She would fall into a depression and stay home alone, day after day.

With the isolation and physical inactivity, Paula gained weight, her muscles cramped, her joints got stiff, and her sleep deteriorated. Feeling weak and fatigued, Paula's pain got worse and she lost touch with the things she loved to do, such as taking quiet walks in the woods and enjoying coffee with friends.

Reluctant to try yoga because she feared it would only make everything worse, Paula finally signed up for our Mindful Yoga class to appease her mental health counselor, who had recommended it multiple times. To her surprise, she discovered that the posture practice was not just tolerable, it was soothing and invigorating. But she was even more surprised that the combination of daily meditation and the informal practices—such as riding the waves of breath and noticing the mind's story in the midst of activities—helped even more. Halfway through the course she said, "To me, simple being is a little sanctuary inside that I can duck into anytime, and it's untouchable—nothing can take it away."

During the remaining weeks of the course, Paula developed insight into the rut she'd stumbled into over and over. She saw clearly that her tendency to overdo activities was the initial step that led to downward spirals. She discovered that if she just persisted in her posture, breathing, and meditation practices; committed to not overdoing tasks; and also committed to leaving her apartment at least once a day, she didn't drift into these ruts.

"I'm getting good at seeing when I'm pushing myself too far," Paula said, "how it amplifies my pain, and I start having all kinds of negative thoughts and feelings. When that happens, I now know how to steer myself back on course. This makes a big difference for my pain, sleep, and overall mood. In fact, I'm feeling a kind of peace I've never experienced before."

Mindful Yoga Review

Hopefully you have now become more familiar with simple being—this stable, undeniable core of yourself. Simple being is not only a refuge that is always *with* you—simple being *is* you, your sense of "I," your very being, your awareness. Just as a diamond may have five distinct facets, simple being has different aspects—including awareness, love, acceptance, and riding the waves—yet is not separate from them. As you continue to explore simple being, you will gradually discover more about this treasure at the center.

Within awareness, life presents itself as an ocean upon which countless waves are constantly arising, peaking, and subsiding. Like the wind, some patterns shift quickly, such as our thoughts. Others, like the earth's rotation, change slowly, such as our body's bony structure. The challenge of life is to learn to ride—that is, to skillfully navigate—all these various waves.

Among the most difficult to ride are the waves of pain. But because pain is influenced by many other types of waves, the Mindful Yoga practices (postures, meditation, breath, self-study, keeping company with truth) and their applications to daily life (for example, watching sensations in a nonreactive way) offer many strategies for gradually calming the waves of pain.

> Simple being *is* you, your sense of "I," your very being, your awareness.

This Mindful Yoga program was designed to help you learn to skillfully ride specific wave patterns that clearly influence pain. As a reminder, here are the most important navigational points to guide you in riding the various waves explored in this book:

Breath is a constant companion that both reflects—and can actively shift—your present-moment experience. If you are upset by pain or anything else, your breath becomes agitated, but you can work skillfully with the breath to shift out of that pattern.

Attention is similar to the rudder on a boat—it steers and focuses awareness. When skillfully applied, attention steers you to calmer waters. Unskillful attention can neurologically amplify pain.

Stress arises when you perceive something as threatening in some way, and staying stressed strongly drives waves of pain. Pay attention to whether you are battling versus riding the waves of stress.

The mind's story interprets events nearly all the time, and our attention tends to become fascinated by and to fuse with this interpretation. Fusion leads to confusion, which can worsen your pain. Notice that the mind's narratives about events are not the same as the events themselves. This is critical because modern neuroscience confirms that buying into negative mental narratives amplifies how pain sensations are processed in the brain.

Pain happens when the brain perceives a bodily threat or damage. However, that perception is strongly influenced by how you relate to sensations—especially those experienced as painful—and how sensations are affected by your thoughts, emotions, and actions. Though challenging, shifting how you relate to sensations is very therapeutic. Yoga practices help generate this shift.

Emotions infuse life with its many flavors, and yet emotions can become turbulent and powerfully exacerbate pain. Yoga practices are effective for increasing emotional well-being, which can greatly reduce pain.

Fatigue is inevitable at times and worsens in the context of chronic pain. Yoga often relieves fatigue because the practices lead to feeling both deeply relaxed and invigorated. When fatigue improves, pain usually does too.

Making the Most of What You've Learned

Whenever you've completed a rather lengthy process of learning new material, it's valuable to reflect on what stands out as most useful from what you've learned. Please reflect on these two questions and write your answers below:

What are the three most important things you have learned from this course?

_____

_____

_____

_____

_____

How will you make sure you don't lose sight of what you've learned?

_____

_____

_____

_____

_____

Eight weeks is clearly not enough time to master yoga. But hopefully you've experienced that daily practice ensures that your boat for this journey has a sturdy and well-balanced hull that can reliably navigate toward the harbor of greater resiliency and pain relief.

At this point, you may want to set the book aside as you continue to practice on your own, with the audio recordings and videos helping to guide your home practice. During this time, notice what happens as you continue to apply what has really stuck with you from the Mindful Yoga program.

If, after several weeks (or months) you find that you are struggling with chronic pain, we suggest you reread this book from beginning to end. Based on our own experiences of studying yoga, it's very likely that you will discover and absorb more from this book the second time around. Some topics or practices that seemed less relevant or accessible to you during your first read will probably become clearly applicable the next time around.

In the meantime, here are some suggestions to make the most of what you've learned so far.

Make the Practices Your Own

Until this point, each chapter has provided recommendations for which practices to do and how often to do them. Now it's time for you to choose the practices that are most meaningful for you currently. You might want to sketch out an initial formal yoga practice plan, including which practices you'll do, how often, at what times of the day, and for how long. It's best to include some mixture of yoga postures, breathing, and meditation practices.

We recommend doing a formal practice every day—even if it's just for fifteen or twenty minutes. Ideally, sit in meditation every day, and practice gentle yoga postures at least three times a week. If you're interested in taking a yoga class in your community, see our guide to *Finding a Skilled Yoga Teacher*, available at http://www.newharbinger.com/43287.

> Now it's time for you to choose the practices that are most meaningful for you currently.

Also consider emphasizing various informal practices, such as noticing stress reactions in daily life, observing the difference between the mind's stories and actual events, or applying different yoga-based tools for working with sensations. Then after trying out that plan for a month or so, review it and decide whether it's working well or if you want to alter your practice plan. Remember, there are no rights or wrongs in making the practice your own—it's up to you to discover which practices serve you best for improving your pain, fatigue, mood, and overall quality of life.

Explore Deepening Your Meditation Practice

Types of meditation vary according to the particular qualities of attention that each cultivates. In this book, you've seen the guided meditation practices evolve from Week 1 through Week 7. With each week, your focusing ability was further developed to become both clearer and more flexible, so that your attention could extend to many other aspects of experience—hearing, sensing, emotions, and observing thoughts. At the same time, a type of open-focus, nondirected choiceless awareness skill was developed in the meditation practice, especially by resting into simple being while allowing all other aspects of experience—sounds, sensations, emotions, thoughts—to continue as they are, neither following them with attention nor withholding attention from them (Krishnamurti 1992).

For readers who are interested in further deepening their meditation practice, we have included an additional guided meditation recording: Breath Through Choiceless Awareness. You can access it at http://www.newharbinger.com/43287. Give it a try when you feel ready.

Be Accountable

Be sure to ask yourself, "What might get in the way of doing my practices?" This is important to consider so that you can plan ahead for the inevitable hurdle. For example, if you're the kind of person who does better when you are following a structured plan, such as what's outlined in the chapters of this book, then devising your own plan and actually trying to follow it may be quite challenging. If that's the case, what could bolster your commitment to practice? Maybe sharing your plan with a close friend or partner and asking them to remind you of your commitment could help.

Or perhaps your initial plan is unrealistic and too demanding for you right now, and you need to start with an easier plan. Recognize that "success builds upon success." It's best to start simple and feel good about your ability to follow your plan, rather than to devise a challenging plan and feel bad about falling short.

Last, it's a good idea to schedule time for a brief weekly check-in with yourself about your practice plan. For example, on Saturday or Sunday mornings spend five to ten minutes reviewing how much you practiced during the week, and consider how well your plan is working.

See Setbacks as Offering New Learning Opportunities

Setbacks of some sort are inevitable in life, and they often occur when you're dealing with pain flares and other unpredictable waves. So it's best to assume that, from time to time, something will happen that will make you hurt more, feel more tired, get upset, or become confused. Each setback, though difficult to face, also offers an opportunity to learn how to better ride the waves. Here are some steps to follow when you realize you're in the middle of a setback:

1. **Pause, notice, and feel.** Identify what is going on for you at this point—changes in pain, fatigue, emotions, thoughts, activities—and how you are reacting.

2. **Practice resiliency.** Extend kindness toward yourself and use whichever of the yoga tools work best for you.

3. **Briefly review the situation leading up to the setback.** Were there any warning signs that might have been important in leading to this setback, such as changes in the weather, new work-related demands, or other factors? Is there something to be learned from what happened that could help you cope better the next time a similar situation arises?

Launch Yourself on Every Wave

One of the most powerful tools for pain relief is love, which is considered by yogic teachings to be the central defining virtue of human experience. Our Mindful Yoga program encourages you to broaden your relationship to love—including noticing and having compassion for the deep survival instinct that drives your reactivity to events that seem "wrong," such as difficult sensations. Can you remember to keep coming back, to return with kindness to everything that is actually here, including the ease of simple being?

As cited in Week 1, the great American writer Henry David Thoreau was strongly influenced by yogic texts, and his advice was to "launch yourself on every wave." Riding the waves is a lifetime curriculum. Our wish for you is that waves of difficult sensations become but momentary currents in the ocean of this precious life.

Mindful Yoga Posture Practices

We offer two options for the Mindful Yoga posture practices:

- **Up-and-Down Sequence**—includes postures done lying down and standing

- **Seated-and-Standing Sequence**—includes postures done sitting in a chair and standing

Both options are beneficial and based on traditional yoga posture practices. The Up-and-Down Sequence involves getting down to the floor and coming back up again, so it may not be appropriate for those who have been very sedentary and/or are unable to do this comfortably or safely. If you are able to lie down on a mat on the floor, please do so. If you're not able to lie down on the floor, it's fine to do the lying-down poses in the Up-and-Down Sequence in your bed. However, if doing postures lying down feels like a strain, you may prefer to practice the Seated-and-Standing sequence.

While it's fine to try both sequences, we recommend that you pick the sequence that feels most comfortable for you and practice that one.

A towel or blanket can be a useful prop when folded into a support, for example, for your lower back when you are sitting in a chair or for your head if your chin pokes up when you are lying down. Optional props include a yoga strap (or bathrobe belt or old necktie), a yoga block, and a small pillow.

For both sequences, new postures will be added to your practice at regular intervals. This method will give you a chance to practice familiar postures while slowly increasing your capacity. As the weeks go by, new points of emphasis will be introduced as well.

Regardless of which sequence you are practicing, *please always begin with Three-Part Breath and end with Relaxation*. Please use the guided audio and/or video instructions at http://www.newharbinger.com/43287 to support your practice.

> **Feel free to let each body part enjoy its fullest range of motion, even if the movement becomes asymmetrical.**

Up-and-Down Sequence pages 137-183

Week 1 Postures 1–8

Weeks 2 & 3 Postures 1–13

Weeks 4 & 5 Postures 1–19

Weeks 6 & 7 Postures 1–26

Seated-and-Standing Sequence pages 169-194

Week 1 Postures 1–6

Weeks 2 & 3 Postures 1–10

Weeks 4 & 5 Postures 1–15

Weeks 6 & 7 Postures 1–20

Up-and-Down Sequence

Week 1 Practice

Postures 1–8

Postures 1 through 8 are done on your back with knees bent and arms by your sides.

Please use the guided audio and/or video instructions at http://www.newharbinger.com/43287 to support your practice.

1. Centering and Breathing

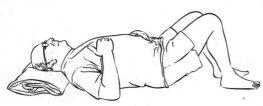

Figure 1.1a

Rest your palms on your lower belly and turn your attention to your breath.

Feel the movement of your breath, just as it is.

Practice Three-Part Breath for 5 cycles (see page 29 to review the instructions; see also **Figure 1.1a**).

Remember: Your breath will let you know if you need to reduce your effort in the postures. If you find that your breath is compromised in any way as you move through a posture, give yourself permission to do a little less until your breath flows comfortably.

2. Arms Overhead

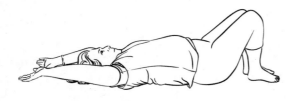

Figure 2.1a

Inhale as you extend your arms up toward the sky and then toward the floor only as far as is comfortable (see **Figure 2.1a**).

Exhale as you bring your arms back to rest by your sides.

Repeat for a few breath cycles.

Remember: Without holding your breath, explore synchronizing your movement with your breath so that the length of your breath matches the length of your movement.

3. Pelvic Tilts

Inhale as you round your belly and tilt your pelvis forward to feel your low back arch away from the floor (see **Figure 3.1a**).

Exhale as you hug your belly toward your spine (like zipping up too-tight jeans) and press your lower back into the floor.

Inhale as you soften your belly and allow your low back to arch up slightly away from the floor.

Continue for a few breath cycles.

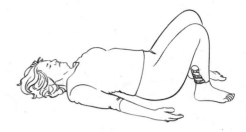

Figure 3.1a

4. Pelvic Tilts with Arms Overhead

Inhale as you soften your belly, tilt your pelvis forward, and lengthen your arms up toward the sky and in the direction of your ears (see **Figure 4.1a**).

Exhale as you hug your belly toward your spine and bring your arms back down by your hips.

Repeat several times.

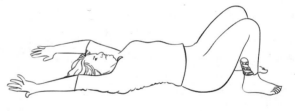

Figure 4.1a

Remember: Without shortening your breath, allow the length of your breath to match the length of your movement. Notice sensations, emotions, and thoughts that occur without judging or trying to make anything different.

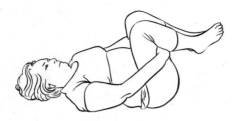

Figure 5.1a

5. Knees to Belly

Take an easy breath in.

As you exhale, draw your right knee in toward your belly. Feel free to hold your leg behind your thigh, or use a strap to hold your leg.

Pause for a few breaths. With each exhale, allow your thigh to come a little closer to your belly. Each time you inhale, allow your thigh to move slightly away from your belly.

Release and repeat with your left leg.

Next, if you'd like, try drawing both knees to your chest at the same time—feeling free to open your thighs wider if that is more comfortable (see **Figure 5.1a**).

Remember: Notice the sensations that arise, whether sensations of fluidity or of restriction or both. Notice if your mind has different responses to the various sensations.

6. *Universal Legs*

Exhale as you hug your right knee toward your belly, holding your leg wherever it is comfortable (see **Figure 6.1a**).

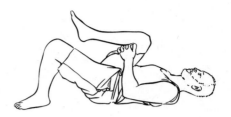

Figure 6.1a

Make circles with your right ankle in both directions to fully explore the range of motion.

Inhale as you lengthen your leg toward the sky (see **Figure 6.2a**).

Exhale as you bend your knee.

Repeat a few times.

Next, leave your right leg in the up position, then flex and point your foot a few times.

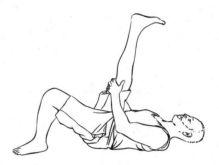

Figure 6.2a

Pause for a few breaths with your foot flexed, your heel reaching toward the ceiling and your sacrum pressing into the floor.

Bend your knee and return your right foot to the ground.

Pause and notice any reactions.

Repeat with your left leg.

Remember: If it's difficult to hold your leg, try using a strap. Or just rest your arms on the floor as you move your leg. As always, challenge yourself but don't strain. Just do the best you can.

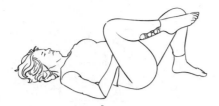

Figure 7.1a

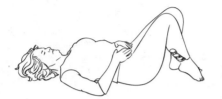

Figure 7.2a

7. Fishing for Salmon

With knees bent, engage your low belly, like zipping up too-tight jeans.

Inhale as you draw your right thigh in toward your belly (see **Figure 7.1a**).

Exhale as you slowly lower your right foot until your toes just barely touch the ground (see **Figure 7.2a**).

Inhale your right knee back toward your belly.

Exhale, engaging your deep belly muscles, as you lower your right foot until your toes lightly touch the floor.

Continue to move with your breath for a couple of rounds.

Repeat with the left leg.

Remember: If you'd like more challenge, keep both thighs near your belly as you move one leg at a time toward the floor.

8. Lake Mudra

Inhale as you extend your left arm up and back toward your ears and your right leg out, hovering just above the floor (see **Figure 8.1a**).

Exhale as you return to the starting position.

Inhale as you extend your right arm and left leg, lengthening across the diagonal.

Exhale as you return to the starting position.

Continue for several rounds, inhaling to extend across the diagonal and exhaling to return.

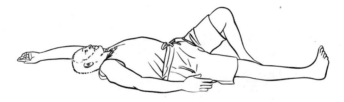

Figure 8.1a

Remember: Be sure to engage your low belly, drawing it in toward your spine to stabilize your pelvis, without restricting your breath. For more challenge, pause in the extended position while keeping your breath flowing comfortably.

Weeks 2 & 3 Practice

Postures 1–13

Practice postures 1 through 8 from Week 1. Postures 9 through 13 are done in a tabletop position, with hands under shoulders and knees under hips.

Please use the guided audio and/or video instructions at http://www.newharbinger.com/43287 to support your practice.

9. Supple Spine Flow

Inhale as you lift and extend your breastbone toward the wall in front of you and reach your tailbone to the wall behind you (see **Figure 9.1a**).

Exhale as you relax your tailbone down and release your head toward the floor.

Continue articulating your spine for a few breaths, synchronizing the movement with your breath.

Inhale as you lengthen your breastbone forward and tailbone back.

Exhale as you relax your tailbone and move your buttocks toward your heels (see **Figure 9.2a**).

After several cycles, pause with your buttocks as close to your heels as comfortable and relax your head toward the floor. Stack palms or fists and rest your forehead on your hands.

Breathe into your back body.

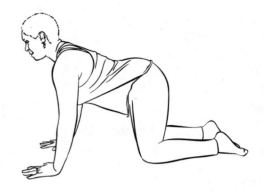

Figure 9.1a

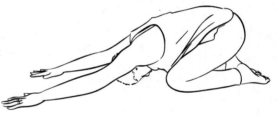

Figure 9.2a

Remember: If your wrists are uncomfortable, come onto your fists or forearms. For sensitive knees, place a pillow or folded towel under them. Avoid pressing into the floor with your hands when your head and tailbone are dropped—don't strongly round your back.

10. Balancing Table

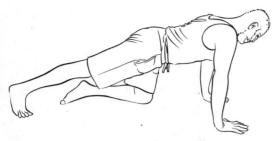

Figure 10.1a

With a neutral spine, press your palms into the floor and hug your belly to your spine.

Step your right leg back with toes tucked under (see **Figure 10.1a**).

Inhale as you lift your right leg up parallel with the floor, keeping your knee and your toes pointing to the ground (see **Figure 10.2a**).

Extend your left arm up by your ear, thumb pointing up (see **Figure 10.3a**). Maintain strength in your belly as you lengthen across the diagonal.

After a few breaths, return your hand and knee to the floor. Relax your head and let your tailbone be heavy. Breathe into your back.

Repeat on the other side.

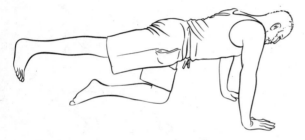

Figure 10.2a

Remember: If this is too hard, lift just the leg or arm, rather than both.

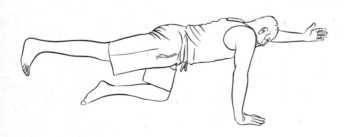

Figure 10.3a

11. Plank Progression

Lower your forearms to the ground, with your elbows under your shoulders. Interlace your fingers and create a tripod of support.

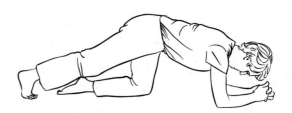

Figure 11.1a

Engage the muscles of your low belly.

Draw your shoulders back and down.

Press your forearms into the ground to engage your arms and chest.

Step your right leg back, toes tucked under, resting on the mat (see **Figure 11.1a**).

Balance your weight evenly in both arms.

Lift your right leg up to the height of your hip, toes and knee facing down (see **Figure 11.2a**).

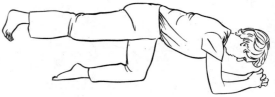

Figure 11.2a

Extend your tailbone toward your heels, press into the ground with your forearms, and keep your belly strong.

Take a few easy breaths then return your right knee to the floor.

Repeat with the left leg.

Remember: To increase the challenge, explore stepping both legs back with the toes tucked under (see **Figure 11.3a**). Find the point of challenge without strain.

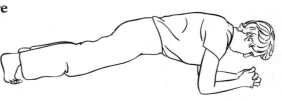

Figure 11.3a

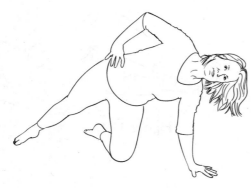

Figure 12.1a

12. Side Plank with Arm Circles

Extend your right leg back, toes tucked under, reaching back through the heel.

Place the inside edge of your right foot on the mat.

Shift your left foot out toward the left side of the mat.

Bring your weight into your left palm and left knee (see **Figure 12.1a**).

Inhale your right arm out and up, so that your right shoulder stacks over your left shoulder and your right arm reaches up.

Make big circles with your right arm, as if it was the hand of a large clock, exploring the range of motion of your right shoulder (see **Figure 12.2a**).

Switch the direction of your circle for a few rounds.

Return to tabletop position and repeat on the other side.

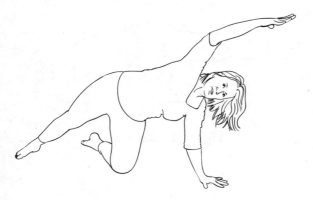

Figure 12.2a

13. Child's Pose

Bring your buttocks back toward your heels as far as comfortably possible.

Stack your palms or fists and rest your forehead on your hands (see **Figure 13.1a**). If you prefer, rest your forehead on a rolled towel, firm pillow, or a yoga block—just be sure your head is supported and not hanging.

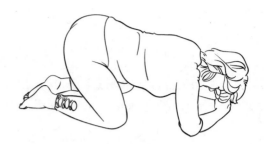

Figure 13.1a

Feel free to open your thighs wider to make room for your body if that's more comfortable.

Breathe into your back body and notice any movement in response to the breath.

Continue for a few breath cycles, inviting a sense of letting go.

Remember: If this pose is not comfortable, try turning it upside down: lie on your back and hug your knees into your chest to stretch out your back.

Weeks 4 & 5 Practice

Postures 1–20

Practice postures 1 through 13 from Weeks 1, 2, and 3. Postures 14 through 20 are done standing with a chair nearby.

Please use the guided audio and/or video instructions at http://www.newharbinger. com/43287 to support your practice.

14. Mountain Pose

Stand tall with your feet hip-distance apart and the four corners of your feet rooting into the ground (see **Figure 14.1a**).

Energize your legs, as if you were a tree drawing up nutrients from the soil.

Release your tailbone down toward the floor, lengthening your back waist.

Gently draw your lower belly in and up, and lift your rib cage up out of your pelvis.

Relax your shoulders down away from your ears.

Extend the top of your head up toward the ceiling, lengthening your spine.

Let your chin be parallel to the ground, neither lifted nor tucked.

Gaze softly toward the horizon, with your shoulders, throat, and face relaxed.

Take several slow, easy breaths, filling and emptying your lungs completely.

Remember: Feel yourself as strong and stable as a mountain. Sense the simultaneous downward and upward energies rooting your legs and lifting your spine.

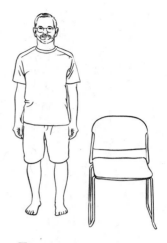

Figure 14.1a

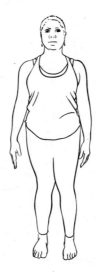

Figure 15.1a

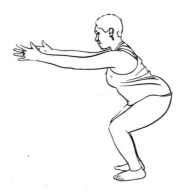

Figure 15.2a

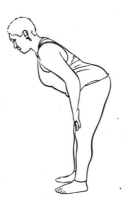

Figure 15.3a

15. Chair Flow

Stand tall in Mountain pose (see **Figure 15.1a**).

Inhale as you sweep your arms forward to the horizon, hinge at your hips, bend your knees, and extend your bottom down as if sitting in a chair (see **Figure 15.2a**). This is called Chair pose.

Exhale as you bring your hands to your thighs and straighten your legs a bit, keeping length in your spine (see **Figure 15.3a**).

Inhale as you float your arms forward, bend your knees, and draw your bottom back into Chair pose (see **Figure 15.2a**).

Exhale as you root into your feet, straighten your legs and body, and stand back into Mountain pose (see **Figure 15.1a**).

Continue for several cycles, letting the heat build.

Remember: Keep your thighs parallel so your knees don't collapse into each other. Make sure you can see your toes when the knees are bent. If not, stick your bottom farther back. Feel free to rest whenever you like.

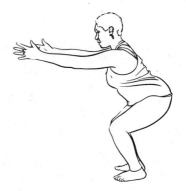

Figure 15.2a

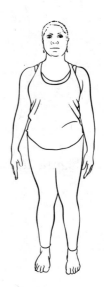

Figure 15.1a

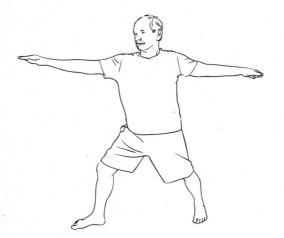

Figure 16.1a

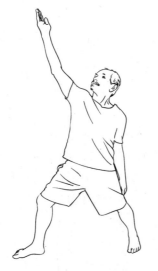

Figure 16.2a

16. Warrior Two Flow

Stand in a wide-legged stance.

Rotate the toes of your right foot 90 degrees to the right.

Rotate the toes of your left foot about 15 degrees to the right. Press gently into your left heel.

Inhale as you extend your arms to the sides while lengthening your spine upward.

Exhale as you bend your right knee so it is above your right heel (see **Figure 16.1a**).

Inhale as you straighten your right knee.

Bend and straighten your knee a few times.

Pause with your right knee bent for a few breaths. Be sure that you have not bent your knee so deeply that you can't see your toes.

Inhale as you extend your right arm up toward the ceiling and relax your left arm down by your left leg (see **Figure 16.2a**).

Exhale as you sweep your right arm out and down to rest your right hand on your right thigh. At the same time, extend your left arm up by your ear (see **Figure 16.3a**).

Moving with your breath, continue this pinwheeling of your arms, keeping your lower body strong and stable.

Repeat on the other side.

Remember: Keep your back leg straight rather than letting the knee collapse. Check that the bent knee tracks directly toward the second toe and doesn't drop inward. If your breath is compromised doing this flow, feel free to do less movement and/or take rest breaks. You will build strength and stamina over time.

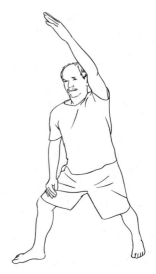

Figure 16.3a

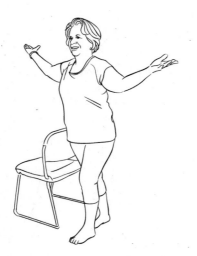

Figure 17.1a

17. Tightrope

Stand in Mountain pose.

Inhale as you extend your arms out to the sides at shoulder height.

Exhale as you soften your shoulders, elbows, and wrists.

Steady your gaze at a point on the horizon.

Shift the weight of your body into your right leg, keeping your hips steady.

Take a baby step forward with your left foot.

If this feels steady, move your left foot closer to your right foot (see **Figure 17.1a**).

If still steady, step your left heel directly in front of your right foot—like walking on a tightrope. If this is too difficult, widen the distance between your feet—like walking a plank.

Shift your weight forward into your left foot, lifting your right heel.

Shift your weight back into your right foot.

Practice slowly shifting your weight from your front foot to your back foot.

For more challenge, step your left foot *behind* your right foot.

When you're ready, step back into Mountain pose, then repeat with your right foot stepping forward.

Remember: Check in with your balance with each step before you progress. Always feel free to rest when necessary. Notice all of the small changes inherent in finding your balance.

18. Tree

Stand in Mountain pose.

Distribute your body weight evenly on both legs and extend the top of your head up.

Root down through your right leg and pick up your left heel, keeping the ball of your foot on the floor.

Turn your left knee out slightly to the left as you slide the sole of your left foot against your right ankle. For more challenge, pick up your left foot and place the sole anywhere along the inside of your right leg—except don't press it against your knee.

Bring one or both palms together at your heart center (see **Figure 18.1a**).

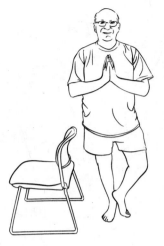

Figure 18.1a

Explore extending your arms up overhead.

Keep your shoulders relaxed and down away from your ears.

Gaze softly at a fixed spot on the horizon.

Extend up through the top of your head as you root down through your right leg and foot. Touch your toe back to the earth anytime you need to, or touch the wall or a chair for support (see **Figure 18.2a**).

Repeat on the other side.

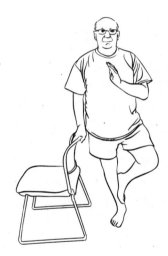

Figure 18.2a

Remember: If you lose your balance, take a breath and try again. Every time your body finds balance, even for a moment, it gets better at balancing.

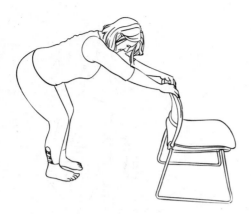

Figure 19.1a

19. Puppy on the Chair

Stand behind your chair with your hands resting on the chair back, about shoulder-width apart.

Hinge at your hips and walk your legs back, so your arms and spine can lengthen.

Keep your knees slightly bent so that your spine stays long and your back doesn't round (see **Figure 19.1a**).

Hug your low belly to your spine to support your low back.

Breathe into the back of your body.

When you're ready, walk your legs back toward the chair and unfold from your hips as you straighten up slowly.

Remember: Find out how far back is comfortable for you. As you become stronger and more flexible, this position may change.

Weeks 6 & 7 Practice

Postures 1–26

Practice postures 1 through 19 from Weeks 1, 2, 3, and 4. Postures 20 through 23 are done with your belly down on the floor.

Please use the guided audio and/or video instructions at http://www.newharbinger. com/43287 to support your practice.

20. Baby Cobra

Lie on your belly, bend your elbows, stack your palms, and rest your forehead on the back of your hands.

Take a few easy breaths and notice where the breath moves.

Next, place your arms down along your sides, palms down.

Rest your forehead or chin on the ground.

Root the front of your pelvis into the ground and extend your legs back, pressing the tops of your feet down. Try not to squeeze your buttocks.

Inhale as you lift up your head, shoulders, and chest (see **Figure 20.1a**).

Exhale as you soften your effort a bit.

Continue for a few breaths. The lifting and softening with your breath may be very small movements. Just try to feel the movement of breath and how it impacts your experience.

When you're done, release back to the ground and rest, supporting your head on the back of your stacked hands if you like.

Take a full easy breath and notice where your breath travels after the backbend.

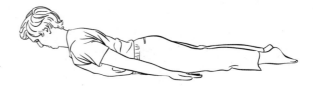

Figure 20.1a

Remember: Keep energy moving down your legs. Only lift your head, shoulders, and chest as high as is comfortable—you may not rise very much, and that's fine. Your strength will build over time. Be sure to keep the back of your neck long, so you're not just lifting and lowering your head, you're using—and cultivating—your back muscles to lift your body.

21. Sphinx

Place your elbows under your shoulders so your forearms are parallel and your palms rest on the ground (see **Figure 21.1a**).

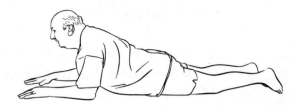

Figure 21.1a

Press the front of your pelvis into the floor.

Lengthen your legs back and press the tops of your feet into the ground.

Shrug your shoulders back and down.

Root down through your pubic bone, and bring your attention to your spine.

Invite each vertebrae, in turn, to extend forward and up.

Lengthen up through the top of your head.

Continue to lengthen back through your legs.

Root your forearms into the ground as you explore the action of pulling the floor toward you isometrically.

Breathe into your back, belly, and chest for several breaths.

When you are ready to release, open your elbows out to the sides and pull the floor toward you with your hands to lengthen your spine.

Rest on your belly for several breaths, head supported on stacked palms.

Remember: Feel how and where the breath moves after a backbend.

22. Locust Flow

Lie on your belly, legs parallel behind you as you bend your elbows out to the sides and stack your palms. Rest your forehead, chin, or cheek on the back of your hands (see **Figure 22.1a**).

Press the front of your pelvis into the ground.

Inhale, stillness.

Exhale as you lift your legs and spread them apart, keeping your knees straight (see **Figure 22.2a**).

Inhale, stillness.

Exhale as you close your legs together and return them to the ground.

Repeat 3 times.

Inhale, stillness.

Exhale as you lift your legs with knees straight, rotate the toes away with *heels together*, and spread the legs apart (see **Figure 22.3a**).

Inhale, stillness.

Exhale as you close your legs together, straighten them, and return them to the ground.

Repeat 3 times.

Inhale, stillness.

Exhale as you lift your legs with knees straight, rotate toes inward with *heels out*, and spread the legs apart (see **Figure 22.4a**).

Inhale, stillness.

Exhale as you close your legs together, straighten them, and return them to the ground.

Repeat 3 times.

Remember: Lift only as high as you can without struggle.

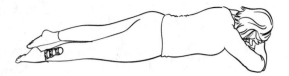

Figure 22.1a

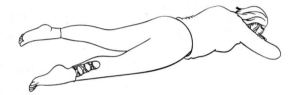

Figure 22.2a

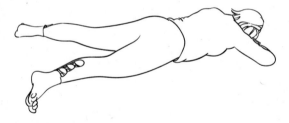

Figure 22.3a

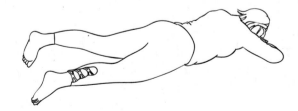

Figure 22.4a

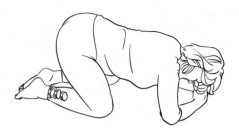

Figure 23.1a

23. *Child's Pose*

From a hands-and-knees position, bring your buttocks back toward your heels as far as comfortably possible.

Stack your palms or your fists (one potato, two potato) and rest your forehead on your hands (see **Figure 23.1a**).

Feel free to open your thighs wider to make room for your body if that's more comfortable.

Rest here, inviting your breath to fill your body and noticing where it moves.

Remember: Feel free to cushion wrists or knees. Or turn the posture upside down—lie on your back and hug your knees into your chest to stretch out your back.

Postures 24 through 26 are done on your back with knees bent and arms by your sides.

Please use the guided audio and/or video instructions at http://www.newharbinger .com/43287 *to support your practice.*

24. Bridge

Set your feet hip-width apart and your palms down.

Exhale as you press down with your feet and lift your hips up off the ground.

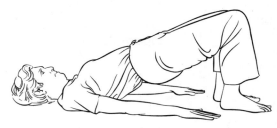

Press your upper arms into the ground to support the lift behind your heart (see **Figure 24.1a**).

Figure 24.1a

Keep your breath flowing comfortably as you linger in the lifted position. Keep your legs parallel— avoid letting your knees knock in or splay out.

When you're done, return your hips to the ground and rest.

Remember: Keep your head straight with your chin in line with the notch between your collarbones. Tilt your chin so it is slightly lower than your forehead—keep the natural curve in your neck.

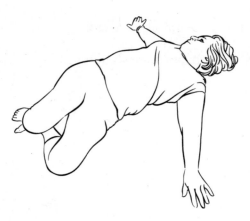

Figure 25.1a

25. Easy Twist

Have one or more pillows or folded towels positioned to the left of your knees.

Set your feet a little wider than hip-width apart.

Extend your arms out to your sides, palms up or down, whichever feels better.

Slowly rock your knees from side to side, keeping your feet on the ground.

Turn your head in the opposite direction of your knees. Keep your movement and breath smooth and easy (see **Figure 25.1a**).

Repeat a few times.

Next, drop your knees to the left, so that they are supported by the pillow or folded towel. Feel free to stack several towels or pillows so that you can comfortably rest both knees onto the support.

Turn your head to the right and linger here for several breaths. On each exhalation, see what you can let go of that you don't need to be holding on to. Breathe into the right side of your body and soften into the twist.

When you're ready, inhale as you bring your legs and head back to center and square yourself off.

Move the pillows or towels to your right side.

On an exhalation, drop your knees onto the supports and turn your head to the left. Linger here for several breaths, as you allow each inhalation to create spaciousness in your left side and each exhalation to soften you into the twist.

Return to the center with bent knees and both feet on the ground, letting your pelvis be very heavy.

Remember: Release the weight of your arms and shoulders into the ground as you gently rotate your spine above and below this area. Be sure your shoulders and shoulder blades stay grounded. Keep the quality of your movements smooth and easy.

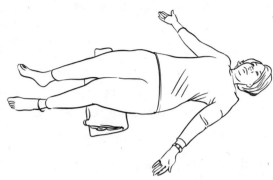

Figure 26.1a

26. Relaxation

Get as comfortable as possible.

Extend your legs long, or bend your knees and support them with a rolled towel or blanket.

Let your hands relax by your sides, palms up or down, whichever position allows you to feel most at ease (see **Figure 26.1a**).

Close your eyes and release the weight of your body into the ground.

Feel the support of the floor holding you up, and—each time you exhale—release your body weight into this support.

Become aware of the pool of sensation that is your body. Greet your body with kindness, and let it be.

Become aware of the waves of your emotional heart. Greet your heart with kindness, and let it be.

Become aware of your thinking mind and the tendencies of your thinking mind. Greet your thinking mind with kindness, and let it be.

For a little while, the invitation is to simply *be*.

Remember: The *undoing* is as important as the doing—learning how to let go and be still is as essential as learning how to move. Give yourself plenty of time for relaxation, at least 7 to 10 minutes, so you can fully benefit from the experience.

Seated-and-Standing Sequence

Week 1 Practice

Postures 1–6

Postures 1 through 6 are done seated in a chair.

Please use the guided audio and/or video instructions at http://www.newharbinger. com/43287 to support your practice.

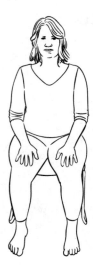

Figure 1.1b

1. Centering and Breathing

Come to a comfortable, dignified seat in a straight-backed chair.

Allow your back to rest against the chair back and your hands to rest in your lap (see **Figure 1.1b**).

For a few moments, observe your breath without trying to change or control it.

Practice Three-Part Breath for 5 cycles (see page 29 to review the instructions).

Remember: If you find that you can't breathe comfortably as you go through the movements, explore doing a little less until your breath is easy and steady.

2. Seated Mountain

Sit slightly forward in your chair with your feet on the ground and hip-width apart.

Tuck your tailbone, as if you are a shy dog.

Next, lift your tailbone, as if you are an excited pup.

Now, find the place in between, where you feel like you are sitting on the base of your pelvis (your sit bones).

Lengthen your spine, lifting your chest and extending the top of your head toward the sky.

Relax your shoulders and neck, and rest your hands on your thighs (see **Figure 2.1b**).

Soften your face and relax your jaw, so that your teeth gently part and your lips barely touch. Soften the inside of your mouth.

Breathe into the stability of Seated Mountain pose.

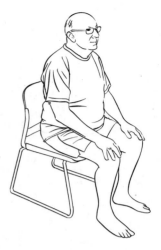

Figure 2.1b

Remember: Sitting upright without the support of the chair back can be surprisingly demanding. If you begin to fatigue and your back starts to round and your chest collapses, scoot back to rest your back against the chair. Keeping good alignment while doing these seated postures is important—so if you need to sit back until you build the strength to sit without support, that's fine.

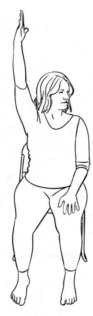

Figure 3.1b

3. Arm and Neck Stretch

Sit tall.

Inhale as you extend your right arm forward and up, and as you turn your head to the left (see **Figure 3.1b**).

Exhale as you return your arm and head back to the starting position.

Repeat on the other side and continue for 5 breaths, alternating arms.

Remember: As always, be sure to challenge yourself but avoid strain. Keep sitting as tall as you can with good alignment throughout the movement.

4. Arching and Bowing Flamingo

Sit tall with palms on thighs.

Inhale as you tilt your pelvis forward so that your pubic bone drops between your thighs and your chest lifts toward the ceiling.

Slide your hands toward your hips.

Look up over your brow, keeping length in back of your neck so that you don't drop your head back (see **Figure 4.1b**).

Exhale as you bring your pelvis, chest, and spine back to neutral alignment.

Relax your chin down toward your chest and slide your hands toward your knees (see **Figure 4.2b**).

Keep your chest lifted so that you don't round your back.

Continue for several breath cycles.

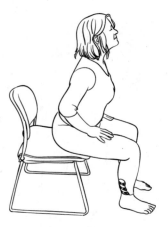

Figure 4.1b

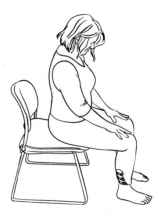

Figure 4.2b

Remember: Be sure not to collapse your chest when your head comes forward. Avoid dropping your head back when you lift your chest toward the ceiling.

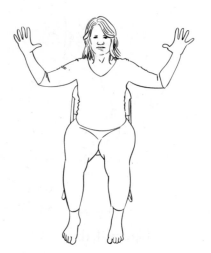

Figure 5.1b

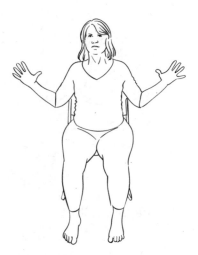

Figure 5.2b: Herculean Arms

5. Herculean Arms

Sit tall.

Inhale as you extend your arms out to the sides, elbows bent and palms forward (see **Figure 5.1b**).

Exhale as you bend your elbows and pull them toward the back of your rib cage (see **Figure 5.2b**).

Emphasize engagement between your shoulder blades.

Pause here for a couple of breaths.

Repeat 3 times.

6. *Leg Lifts*

Sit tall toward the front of your chair.

Hug in your low belly (like zipping up too-tight jeans) while maintaining length in your spine.

Exhale as you extend your right foot forward and up, straightening the leg (see **Figure 6.1b**).

Inhale as you relax your leg back to the floor.

Repeat with your left leg.

Continue for several breaths, alternating legs.

For more challenge, linger with your leg in the up position for several breaths.

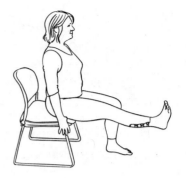

Figure 6.1b

Remember: This can be surprisingly challenging. If your back starts to round and/or your chest begins to collapse, practice maintaining the hug in your low belly and do a little less—perhaps not fully straightening your knee. Lift a little, then rest a little. With practice, your strength will increase—so be patient and persistent, balancing effort and relaxation.

Weeks 2 & 3 Practice

Postures 1–10

Practice postures 1 through 6 from Week 1. Postures 7 through 10 are also done seated in a chair.

Please use the guided audio and/or video instructions at http://www.newharbinger. com/43287 to support your practice.

7. Head Push

Sit tall.

Place your fingertips on your forehead just above the brow (see **Figure 7.1b**).

Inhale as you lengthen your neck upward.

Exhale as you press your fingers into your forehead trying to push your head backward, but don't let it move—gently resist the pressure.

Inhale and soften, exhale and press.

Repeat 3 times.

Explore this pattern with different push points: right then left side of your head just above the ear (see **Figure 7.2b**), and back of your skull just above the neck (see **Figure 7.3b**).

Remember: Strength is built when your muscles resist the push. Resilience is built by softening the muscles between presses.

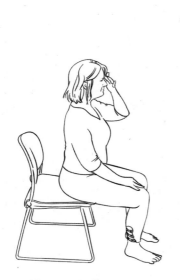

Figure 7.1b

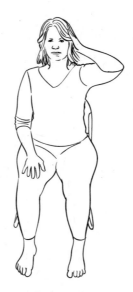

Figure 7.2b

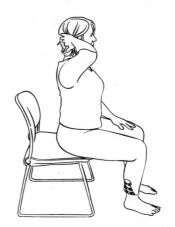

Figure 7.3b

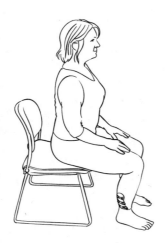

Figure 8.1b

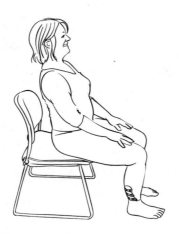

Figure 8.2b

8. Docked Boat

Sit tall toward the front of your chair (see **Figure 8.1b**).

Hug in your low belly without interfering with your breath.

Maintain this engagement in your low belly and lean back slightly in your chair. Be sure to keep your spine long, chest lifted, and shoulders relaxed (see **Figure 8.2b**).

Pause here for a few breaths then return to Seated Mountain pose.

Repeat 2 or 3 times.

Remember: Keep a neutral alignment in your spine as you lean back: if someone were looking at you from the side, your ear, shoulder, and hip would be in alignment. If this strains your back, tilt back less—even just a slight tilt will begin to cultivate strength.

9. Seat Hover

Sit tall (see **Figure 9.1b**).

Engage your low belly and then release.

Engage your low belly as you gently lift the muscles of your pelvic floor (that diamond-shaped area defined by the pubic bone, the tailbone, and each sit bone) in and up, trying not to squeeze your buttocks. Then release.

Inhale as you soften your low belly and your pelvic floor.

Exhale as you draw your low belly toward your spine while lifting the pelvic floor toward the base of your throat.

Repeat 3 times.

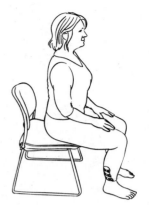

Figure 9.1b

Remember: Do not work so hard at this that your breath becomes choppy. While the action of drawing in the pelvic floor and low belly won't be visible, when these muscles are engaged it may feel a bit like hovering above the seat of the chair.

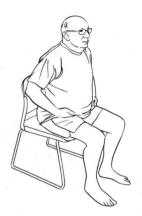

Figure 10.1b

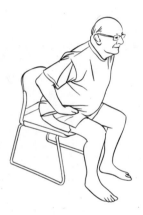

Figure 10.2b

10. "As If" Chair Stands

Sit tall.

Bring your pinkie fingers into the crease where your thigh meets your torso. This is your hip hinge, which is an important landmark for good body mechanics, since learning how to hinge at the hips rather than bend at the waist helps avoid strain on the bones and muscles of your back.

Inhale as you lengthen up from the top of your head (see **Figure 10.1b**).

Exhale as you hinge forward at your hips, pressing your feet into the ground, and activate the muscles of your legs and lower body *as if* you were going to stand (see **Figure 10.2b**).

Relax back into Seated Mountain pose.

Continue several times.

Remember: This practice is a variation of the squat, a staple of strength training routines, that works muscles in the hips, buttocks, legs, and core. It also helps improve balance and coordination.

Weeks 4 & 5 Practice

Postures 1 through 15.

Practice postures 1 through 10 from Weeks 1 and 2. Postures 11 through 15 are done standing with a chair.

Please use the guided audio and/or video instructions at http://www.newharbinger. com/43287 to support your practice.

11. Sun Salutation with a Chair

Stand in Mountain pose about 6 inches behind a chair (see **Figure 11.1b**).

Press the four corners of the feet firmly into the floor. Relax your tailbone, engage your belly, and lift your heart. Feel your breath.

Inhale as you sweep your arms over your head (see **Figure 11.2b**).

Exhale as you fold forward from your hips with knees bent. Land your hands shoulder-width apart on the chair back (see **Figure 11.3b**).

Inhale as you straighten your legs a bit.

Exhale as you bend your knees a bit deeper.

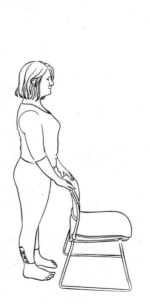

Figure 11.1b

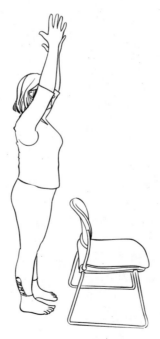

Figure 11.2b

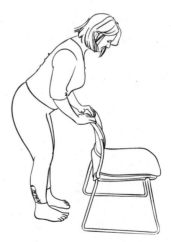

Figure 11.3b

Step the ball of your left foot back behind you as far as is comfortable, keeping the heel lifted. Bend your right knee, being sure that it aligns with your second toe (see **Figure 11.4b**).

Inhale as you lift your heart out of your belly. If you feel steady, lift your arms up by your ears.

Exhale as you place your hands on the chair, step your left foot forward a couple of inches, and step your right foot back beside your left. Bend your knees and extend your tailbone to the back wall, lengthening your spine (see **Figure 11.5b**).

Step your left foot forward toward the chair and slide your right foot back a few inches. Bend your left knee so it is over your ankle and aligned with your toes (see **Figure 11.6b**).

Inhale as you lift your heart, extending your arms toward your ears.

Exhale as you step your right foot forward by the left, bend your knees, and fold over your hips (see **Figure 11.3b**).

Press down through your legs and inhale to unfold your hips, arms reaching overhead (see **Figure 11.2b**).

Exhale into Mountain pose (see **Figure 11.1b**).

Continue for several more cycles.

Remember: Keep your bent knee over your heel and aligned with your toes to avoid straining your knee. Keep your spine long when you fold over your hips—if you feel your back rounding, bend your knees more deeply.

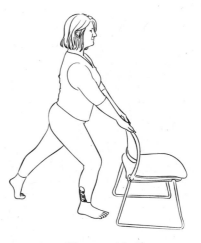

Figure 11.4b

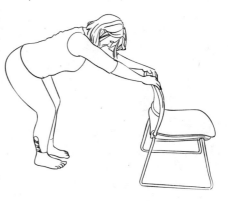

Figure 11.5b

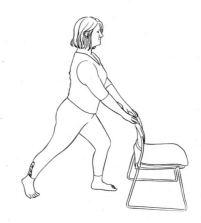

Figure 11.6b

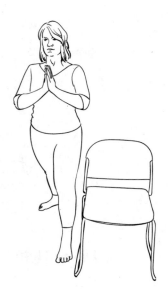

Figure 12.1b

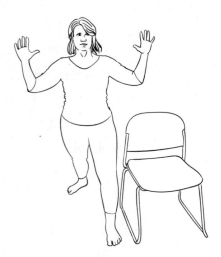

Figure 12.2b

12. Dancing Warrior One

Stand beside the back of your chair.

Anchor into your right leg and rotate your left foot to the left, about 15 degrees.

Take a comfortable step forward with your right leg, knee pointing in the same direction as your toes. Be sure your hips, navel, and right big toe are all facing forward.

Bring your hands together in front of your heart, palms touching (see **Figure 12.1b**).

Press your left heel firmly into the ground to keep your left knee straight.

Inhale as you bend your right knee until it is over your right ankle and open your bent arms out to the sides, drawing your shoulder blades together (see **Figure 12.2b**).

Exhale as you hug your belly to your spine, straighten your right leg, and bring your palms back together.

Repeat 3 times.

Next, inhale as you bend your right knee and open your arms.

Exhale in place and root into your left heel.

With legs steady, inhale and extend your arms overhead (see **Figure 12.3b**).

Exhale as you bend your elbows and bring them down by your hips.

Repeat 3 times.

Try it on the other side.

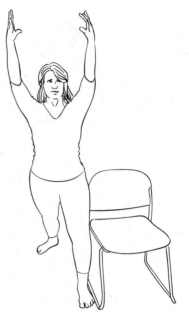

Figure 12.3b

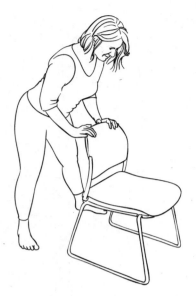

Figure 13.1b

13. A-Stance Forward Fold

Come to a wide-legged stance behind your chair with your feet parallel.

Place your hands on the chair back, shoulder-width apart.

Inhale as you lengthen your spine.

Exhale as you fold forward from the hips, keeping your spine long and your knees soft (see **Figure 13.1b**). Do not bend from the waist. Do not fold so far that your spine begins to round.

Balance the weight of your body between the balls of your feet and your heels.

Inhale as you lengthen from crown to tailbone.

Exhale as you soften through your hips.

Stay here for 3 breaths.

Press into your feet to unfold your hips and return to an upright position.

Remember: Keep your spine in neutral alignment. Although this may be more demanding than rounding or collapsing your spine, maintaining neutral alignment builds strength in the muscles that support your spine. Be sure to come up slowly in case you feel any dizziness.

14. Puppy on the Chair

Stand behind your chair with your hands resting on the chair back, shoulder-width apart.

Hinging at your hips, walk your legs back so your arms and spine can lengthen.

Keep your knees bent so your spine stays long (see **Figure 14.1b**).

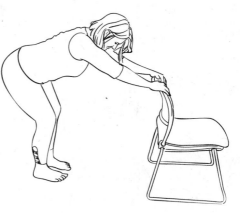

Figure 14.1b

Hug in your low belly to support your back.

Breathe into the back of your body.

When you're ready, walk your legs back toward the chair and come up slowly, unfolding from the hips.

Remember: Find out how far back is comfortable for you. This position may change over time.

15. Tree

Stand tall beside your chair.

Distribute your body weight evenly on both legs and extend the top of your head upward.

Root down through your right leg and pick up your left heel, keeping the ball of your foot on the floor.

Turn your left knee out to the left as you slide the sole of your left foot against your right ankle. For more challenge, pick up your left foot and place the sole anywhere you like along the inside of your right leg—except don't press against your knee.

Bring one or both palms together in front of your heart (see **Figure 15.1b**).

Explore extending your arms up overhead.

Keep your shoulders relaxed and down, away from your ears.

Gaze softly at a fixed spot on the horizon.

Extend up through the top of your head as you root down through your right leg and foot.

Touch your toe down as needed, or touch the wall or a chair for support (see **Figure 15.2b**).

Repeat on the other side.

Remember: If you lose your balance, try again. Every time your body finds balance, even for a moment, it gets better at balancing.

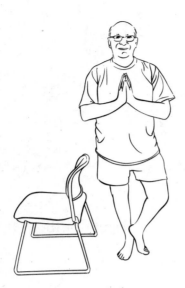

Figure 15.1b

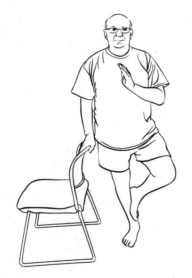

Figure 15.2b

Weeks 6 & 7

Postures 1–20

Practice postures 1 through 15 from Weeks 1 through 5. Postures 16 through 20 are done sitting in a chair.

Please use the guided audio and/or video instructions at http://www.newharbinger. com/43287 to support your practice.

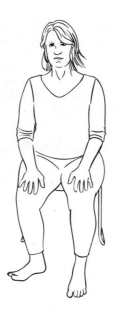

Figure 16.1b

16. *Foot Mopping*

Return to Seated Mountain pose.

Press your right heel into the ground and pivot your foot, rotating the toes and ball of your right foot to the right (see **Figure 16.1b**).

Press the ball of your right foot into the ground and slide it back to the center, as if you were wiping up a spill with a towel under your right foot (see **Figure 16.2b**).

Repeat several times, strengthening the muscles of your foot and ankle.

Repeat with your left foot.

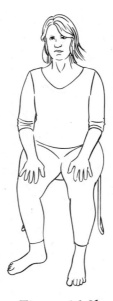

Figure 16.2b

17. Hamstring Strength

Sit tall.

Lengthen your spine and gently hug in the muscles of your low belly. Keep your breath flowing comfortably.

Inhale as you extend your right leg forward with the heel on the ground (see **Figure 17.1b**).

Exhale as you press the heel of your right foot into the ground while sliding the foot back beneath the knee.

Repeat several times, continuing to sit tall without collapsing your spine.

Repeat with your left leg.

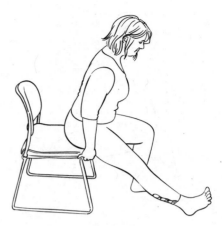

Figure 17.1b

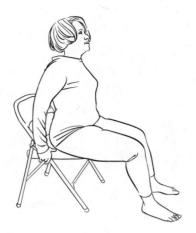

Figure 18.1b

18. Seated Back Bend

Sit tall.

Place one hand on each thigh.

Inhale as you shrug both shoulders back, lift your breastbone toward the ceiling, and draw your shoulder blades together.

Press your palms into your thighs or chair seat to help lift your chest into a backbend (see **Figure 18.1b**).

Do not drop your head back.

Take 3 easy breaths.

On an exhalation, return to Seated Mountain pose.

Practice several times.

Remember: Keep the back of your neck long—avoid dropping your head back.

19. Easy Twist

Sit tall.

Place your right hand on your right thigh and your left hand on top of the right.

Inhale as you lengthen your spine.

Exhale as you rotate your torso to the right (see **Figure 19.1b**). Avoid using your arms, shoulders, or legs to facilitate the twist.

Inhale into the left side of your body, creating space within the twist.

Exhale as you allow something to soften.

Linger here for a few breaths.

Exhale as you return to center.

Repeat to the other side.

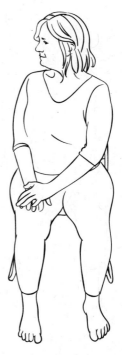

Figure 19.1b

Remember: Keep your rotation in midrange, as it's not advisable to push the twist as far as possible. Also, use the strength of the muscles around your spine to rotate, rather than using your arms to leverage the twist. Strengthening these muscles is important for spinal health.

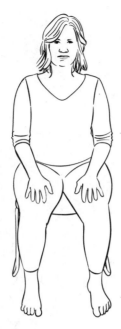

Figure 20.1b

20. Relaxation Pose

Rest your back against the chair back and get as comfortable as possible.

Let your hands rest in your lap in whatever position allows you to feel most at ease

Close your eyes and release the weight of your body.

Take an easy breath in and let it out with a sigh.

Feel the support of the chair and the floor holding you up, and release your body weight into this support each time you exhale.

Become aware of the pool of sensation that is your body. Greet your body with kindness, and let it be.

Become aware of the waves of your emotional heart. Greet your heart with kindness, and let it be.

Become aware of your thinking mind and the tendencies of your thinking mind. Greet your thinking mind with kindness, and let it be.

For a little while, the invitation is to simply be.

Remember: The undoing is as important as the doing—learning how to let go and be still is as essential as learning how to move. Give yourself plenty of time for relaxation, at least 7 to 10 minutes, so you can fully benefit from the experience.

Acknowledgments

From Jim

I am immensely grateful to the very generous enlightened teachers who have illumined my heart and my path, above all to Swami Muktananda and Bhagawan Nityananda, and also to Sri Nisargadatta Maharaj and Joel Morwood. I am deeply thankful to Kimberly, my amazing partner in this work and in life, and I appreciate the support of our children, Grace and Shankara, as we engaged in this labor of love. I thank Jon Kabat-Zinn for his inspirational work, and I am beholden to my mentor, Dr. Francis Keefe, for nourishing the initial development of the Mindful Yoga program. I am grateful to a host of faculty colleagues for their support and also to the wonderful people living with chronic pain who have been receptive to the wisdom of yoga. Last, I thank Carol for encouraging us to write this book and helping greatly in this accomplishment.

From Kimberly

I am eternally grateful for the grace of the yoga tradition and for the awake guidance from Bhagawan Nityananda, Swamis Muktananda and Kripalvananda, Joel Morwood, Lee Lyon, and Micky Singer. I have immense gratitude for the inspiration of Jon Kabat-Zinn and for the confidence and support of Dr. Francis Keefe. Thank you, sweet Jimbo, for being my best friend, husband, colleague, teacher, and student. The pathless path is adorned exquisitely by you and our precious children, Shankara and Grace. Thank you, Carol, for being my soul sister in the myriad dances of life. With great love and respect...

From Carol

I am grateful for the numerous teachers on whose shoulders I stand—in particular the late Esther Myers, a woman of great courage, wisdom, and dignity who dedicated her life to discovering the essence of yoga and exploring how it can be taught clearly, compassionately, and authentically. Deep thanks to my students, who have been among my greatest teachers, and to Jim and Kimberly for being amazing partners on this extraordinary journey. Boundless love to my family for their unwavering support.

How to Get the Accessories for Your Book

We have provided a range of additional helpful materials that are available for free at the publisher's website: http://www.newharbinger.com/43287. If you need help accessing these materials, please visit http://www.newharbinger.com/book-accessories for a step-by-step guide to registering your book. Then you can download these helpful materials onto your computer, tablet, and/or smartphone.

These accessories include bonus chapters, worksheets, guided audios, and streaming video practices, all of which can greatly support your practice of Mindful Yoga and living a vital life. You'll find the following material available:

Bonus Chapters

More About Pain

Finding a Skilled Yoga Teacher

Mindful Yoga Calendars

Week 1 Formal Practice—Beginning Your Mindful Yoga Journey

Week 2 Formal Practice—Riding the Waves of Attention

Week 3 Formal Practice—Riding the Waves of Stress

Week 4 Formal Practice—Riding the Waves of the Mind's Story

Week 5 Formal Practice—Riding the Waves of Pain

Week 6 Formal Practice—Riding the Waves of Emotion

Week 7 Formal Practice—Riding the Waves of Fatigue

Mindful Yoga Journaling Worksheets

Week 1 Keeping the Company of Truth: Riding the Waves of the Breath

Week 2 Keeping the Company of Truth: Riding the Waves of Attention

Week 3 Keeping the Company of Truth: Riding the Waves of Stress

Week 4 Keeping the Company of Truth: Riding the Waves of the Mind's Story

Week 5 Keeping the Company of Truth: Riding the Waves of Pain

Week 6 Keeping the Company of Truth: Riding the Waves of Emotions

Week 7 Keeping the Company of Truth: Riding the Waves of Fatigue

Audio-Guided Breath Practices

Three-Part Breath

Extended Exhalation

Audio-Guided Meditations

I Am

Simple Being, Always Here

Breath and Simple Being

Breath Through Sensing

Breath Through Thoughts

Breath Through Choiceless Awareness

Yoga Nidra

Meditation on Deep-Down Goodness

Audio-Guided Exercise

Emotion Laboratory

Audio-Guided Up-and-Down Posture Practice

Week 1

Weeks 2 & 3

Weeks 4 & 5

Weeks 6 & 7

Weeks 1–3

Weeks 1–5

Weeks 1–7

Audio-Guided Seated-and-Standing Posture Practice

Week 1

Weeks 2 & 3

Weeks 4 & 5

Weeks 6 & 7

Weeks 1–3

Weeks 1–5

Weeks 1–7

Video-Guided Up-and-Down Posture Practice

Week 1

Weeks 2 & 3

Weeks 4 & 5

Weeks 6 & 7

Weeks 1–3

Weeks 1–5

Weeks 1–7

Video-Guided Seated-and-Standing Posture Practice

Week 1

Weeks 2 & 3

Weeks 4 & 5

Weeks 6 & 7

Weeks 1–3

Weeks 1–5

Weeks 1–7

If you're having trouble getting these accessories, just visit http://www.newharbinger.com /book-accessories for a step-by-step guide to registering your book. Then you can download these helpful materials onto your computer, tablet, and/or smartphone.

References

Alshelh, Z., K. K. Marciszewski, R. Akhter, F. Di Pietro, E. P. Mills, E. R. Vickers, C. C. Peck, G. M. Murray, and L. A. Henderson. 2018. "Disruption of Default Mode Network Dynamics in Acute and Chronic Pain States." *NeuroImage: Clinical* 17: 222–231. https://doi.org/10.1016/j.nicl.2017.10.019.

American Psychological Association. 2017. *Stress in America: Coping with Change.* Stress in America Survey. Accessed February 20, 2019. https://www.apa.org/news/press/releases/stress/2016/coping-with-change.pdf.

Apkarian, A. V., J. A. Hashmi, and M. N. Baliki. 2011. "Pain and the Brain: Specificity and Plasticity of the Brain in Clinical Chronic Pain." *Pain* 152: S49–64.

Baer, R. A. 2003. "Mindfulness Training as a Clinical Intervention: A Conceptual and Empirical Review." *Clinical Psychology: Science and Practice* 10: 125–143.

Baker, K. S., S. Gibson, N. Georgiou-Karistianis, R. M. Roth, and M. J. Giummarra. 2016. "Everyday Executive Functioning in Chronic Pain: Specific Deficits in Working Memory and Emotion Control, Predicted by Mood, Medications, and Pain Interference." *Clinical Journal of Pain* 32: 673–80. https://doi.org/10.1097/ajp.0000000000000313.

Bayer, T. L., P. E. Baer, and C. Early. 1991. "Situational and Psychophysiological Factors in Psychologically Induced Pain." *Pain* 44: 45–50.

Bayer, T. L., J. H. Coverdale, E. Chiang, and M. Bangs. 1998. "The Role of Prior Pain Experience and Expectancy in Psychologically and Physically Induced Pain." *Pain* 74: 327–31.

Berzin, R. 2019. "A Simple Breathing Exercise to Calm Your Mind & Body." Accessed February 15, 2019. http://www.mindbodygreen.com/0-4386/A-Simple-Breathing-Exercise-to-Calm-Your-Mind-Body.html.

Buffart, L. M., J. G. van Uffelen, I. I. Riphagen, J. Brug, W. van Mechelen, W. J. Brown, and M. J. Chinapaw. 2012. "Physical and Psychosocial Benefits of Yoga in Cancer Patients and Survivors: A Systematic Review and Meta-Analysis of Randomized Controlled Trials." *BMC Cancer* 12: 559.

Busch, V., W. Magerl, U. Kern, J. Haas, G. Hajak, and P. Eichhammer. 2012. "The Effect of Deep and Slow Breathing on Pain Perception, Autonomic Activity, and Mood Processing: An Experimental Study." *Pain Medicine* 13: 215–28.

Butler, D. S., and L. Moseley. 2013. *Explain Pain.* 2nd ed. Adelaide, Australia: Noigroup Publications.

Carlson, L. E., and S. N. Garland. 2005. "Impact of Mindfulness-Based Stress Reduction (MBSR) on Sleep, Mood, Stress and Fatigue Symptoms in Cancer Outpatients." *International Journal of Behavioral Medicine* 12: 278–85.

Carson, J. W., and K. M. Carson. 2019. Mindful Yoga Professional Training Manual.

Carson, J. W., K. M. Carson, K. M. Gil, and D. H. Baucom. 2004. "Mindfulness-Based Relationship Enhancement." *Behavior Therapy* 35: 471–494.

Carson, J. W., K. M. Carson, K. D. Jones, R. M. Bennett, C. L. Wright, and S. D. Mist. 2010. "A Pilot Randomized Controlled Trial of the Yoga of Awareness Program in the Management of Fibromyalgia." *Pain* 151: 530–9.

Carson, J. W., K. M. Carson, K. D. Jones, L. Lancaster, and S. D. Mist. 2016. "Mindful Yoga Pilot Study Shows Modulation of Abnormal Pain Processing in Fibromyalgia Patients." *International Journal of Yoga Therapy* 26: 93–100. https://doi.org/10.17761/IJYT2016_Research_Carson_Epub.

Carson, J. W., K. M. Carson, K. D. Jones, S. D. Mist, and R. M. Bennett. 2012. "Follow-Up of Yoga of Awareness for Fibromyalgia: Results at 3 Months and Replication in the Wait-List Group." *Clinical Journal of Pain* 28: 804–13.

Carson, J. W., K. M. Carson, L. S. Porter, F. J. Keefe, and V. L. Seewaldt. 2009. "Yoga of Awareness Program for Menopausal Symptoms in Breast Cancer Survivors: Results from a Randomized Trial." *Supportive Care in Cancer* 17: 1301–1309.

Carson, J. W., K. M. Carson, L. S. Porter, F. J. Keefe, H. Shaw, and J. M. Miller. 2007. "Yoga for Women with Metastatic Breast Cancer: Results from a Pilot Study." *Journal of Pain & Symptom Management* 33: 331–41.

Carson, J. W., F. J. Keefe, T. R. Lynch, K. M. Carson, V. Goli, A. M. Fras, and S. R. Thorp. 2005. "Loving-Kindness Meditation for Chronic Low-back pain: Results from a Pilot Trial." *Journal of Holistic Nursing* 23: 1–18.

Cramer, H., R. Lauche, and J. Langhorst. 2013. "Yoga for Depression: A Systematic Review and Meta-Analysis." *Depression and Anxiety* 30: 1,068–1,083.

Davidson, R. J., J. Kabat-Zinn, J. Schumacher, M. Rosenkranz, D. Muller, S. F. Santorelli, F. Urbanowski, A. Harrington, K. Bonus, and J. F. Sheridan. 2003. "Alterations in Brain and Immune Function Produced by Mindfulness Meditation." *Psychosomatic Medicine* 65: 564–70.

Dhruva, A., C. Miaskowski, D. Abrams, M. Acree, B. Cooper, S. Goodman, and F. M. Hecht. 2012. "Yoga Breathing for Cancer Chemotherapy-Associated Symptoms and Quality of Life: Results of a Pilot Randomized Controlled Trial." *Journal of Alternative & Complementary Medicine* 18: 473–9.

Doherty, E. M., R. Walsh, L. Andrews, and S. McPherson. 2017. "Measuring Emotional Intelligence Enhances the Psychological Evaluation of Chronic Pain." *Journal of Clinical Psychology in Medical Settings* 24: 365–375. https://doi.org/10.1007/s10880-017-9515-x.

Doidge, N. 2007. *The Brain That Changes Itself.* New York: Penguin Books.

Eastman-Mueller, H., T. Wilson, A. K. Jung, A. Kimura, and J. Tarrant. 2013. "iRest Yoga-Nidra on the College Campus: Changes in Stress, Depression, Worry, and Mindfulness." *International Journal of Yoga Therapy* 23 (2): 15–24.

Epel, E., J. Daubenmier, J. T. Moskowitz, S. Folkman, and E. Blackburn. 2009. "Can Meditation Slow Rate of Cellular Aging? Cognitive Stress, Mindfulness, and Telomeres." *Annals of the New York Academy of Sciences* 1172: 34–53.

Faulds, S. R. 2005. "A Kripalu Yoga Definition of Enlightenment." *Yoga Bulletin of the Kripalu Yoga Teachers Association* 14: 8–9.

Finan, P. H., B. R. Goodin, and M. T. Smith. 2013. "The Association of Sleep and Pain: An Update and a Path Forward." *Journal of Pain* 14: 1,539–52. https://doi.org/10.1016/j.jpain.2013.08.007.

Garfinkel, M. S., A. Singhal, W. A. Katz, D. A. Allan, R. Reshetar, H. R. Schumacher. 1998. "Yoga-Based Intervention for Carpal Tunnel Syndrome: A Randomized Trial." *JAMA* 280: 1,601–3.

Garfinkel, M. S., H. R. Schumacher, Jr., A. Husain, M. Levy, R. A. Reshetar, N. Full, H. R. J. Schumacher, A. Husain, M. Levy, and R. A. Reshetar. 1994. "Evaluation of a Yoga-Based Regimen for Treatment of Osteoarthritis of the Hands." *Journal of Rheumatology* 21: 2,341–2,343.

Germaine, L. M., and R. R. Freedman. 1984. "Behavioral Treatment of Menopausal Hot Flashes: Evaluation by Objective Methods." *Journal of Consulting and Clinical Psychology* 52(6):1,072–79.

Gilden, D. L., and H. Hancock. 2007. "Response Variability in Attention-Deficit Disorders." *Psychological Science* 18: 796–802. https://doi.org/10.1111/j.1467-9280.2007.01982.x.

Goldberg, D. S., and S. J. McGee. 2011. "Pain as a Global Public Health Priority." *BMC Public Health* 11: 770. https://doi.org/10.1186/1471-2458-11-770.

Goleman, D. J., and G. E. Schwartz. 1976. "Meditation as an Intervention in Stress Reactivity." *Journal of Consulting and Clinical Psychology* 44: 456–466.

Grant, J. A. 2014. "Meditative Analgesia: The Current State of the Field." *Annals of the New York Academy of Sciences* 1307: 55–63.

Hartranft, C. 2003. *The Yoga-Sutra of Patanjali: A New Translation with Commentary.* Boston: Shambala.

Hayes, S. C., V. M. Follett, and M. M. Linehan. 2004. *Mindfulness and Acceptance.* New York: Guilford.

Hayes, S. C., J. B. Luoma, F. W. Bond, A. Masuda, and J. Lillis. 2006. "Acceptance and Commitment Therapy: Model, Processes and Outcomes." *Behaviour Research & Therapy* 44: 1–25.

Hayes, S. C., K. Strosahl, and K. G. Wilson. 1999. *Acceptance and Commitment Therapy: An Experiential Approach to Behavior Change.* New York: Guilford Press.

Holzel, B. K., S. W. Lazar, T. Gard, Z. Schuman-Olivier, D. R. Vago, and U. Ott. 2011. "How Does Mindfulness Meditation Work? Proposing Mechanisms of Action from a Conceptual and Neural Perspective." *Perspectives on Psychological Science* 6: 537–559.

Holzel, B. K., U. Ott, H. Hempel, A. Hackl, K. Wolf, R. Stark, and D. Vaitl. 2007. "Differential Engagement of Anterior Cingulate and Adjacent Medial Frontal Cortex in Adept Meditators and Non-Meditators." *Neuroscience Letters* 421: 16–21.

Institute of Medicine. 2011. *Relieving Pain in America: A Blueprint for Transforming Prevention, Care, Education, and Research.* Washington, D.C.: The National Academies Press.

Irwin, M. R., R. Olmstead, C. Carrillo, N. Sadeghi, J. D. Fitzgerald, V. K. Ranganath, and P. M. Nicassio. 2012. "Sleep Loss Exacerbates Fatigue, Depression, and Pain in Rheumatoid Arthritis." *Sleep* 35: 537–43. https://doi.org/10.5665/sleep.1742.

John, P. J., N. Sharma, C. M. Sharma, and A. Kankane. 2007. "Effectiveness of Yoga Therapy in the Treatment of Migraine Without Aura: A Randomized Controlled Trial." *Headache* 47: 6,54–61.

Kabat-Zinn, J. 1990. *Full Catastrophe Living: Using the Wisdom of Your Body and Mind in Everyday Life.* New York: Delacorte.

Keefe, F. J., M. E. Rumble, C. D. Scipio, L. A. Giordano, and L. M. Perri. 2004. "Psychological Aspects of Persistent Pain: Current State of the Science." *Journal of Pain* 5: 195–211.

Krishnamurti, J. 1992. *Choiceless Awareness.* Ojai, CA.: Krishnamurti Publications of America.

Lazarus, R. S., and S. Folkman. 1984. *Stress, Appraisal, and Coping.* New York: Springer.

Lehrer, P., R. Carr, D. Sargunaraj, and R. Woolfolk. 1994. "Stress Management Techniques: Are They All Equivalent, or Do They Have Specific Effects?" *Biofeedback and Self-Regulation* 19: 353–401.

Maharshi, R. 2000. *Talks with Ramana Maharshi: On Realizing Abiding Peace and Happiness.* Carlsbad, CA: InnerDirections.

Martell, B. A., P. G. O'Connor, R. D. Kerns, W. C. Becker, K. H. Morales, T. R. Kosten, and D. A. Fiellin. 2007. "Systematic Review: Opioid Treatment for Chronic Back Pain: Prevalence, Efficacy, and Association with Addiction." *Annals of Internal Medicine* 146: 116–127.

Martin, S. L., K. L. Kerr, E. J. Bartley, B. L. Kuhn, S. Palit, E. L. Terry, J. L. DelVentura, and J. L. Rhudy. 2012. "Respiration-Induced Hypoalgesia: Exploration of Potential Mechanisms." *Journal of Pain* 13: 755–63.

McCracken, L. M., J. W. Carson, C. Eccleston, and F. J. Keefe. 2004. "Acceptance and Change in the Context of Chronic Pain." *Pain* 109: 4–7.

McCracken, L. M., K. E. Vowles, and C. Eccleston. 2005. "Acceptance-Based Treatment for Persons with Complex, Long-Standing Chronic Pain: A Preliminary Analysis of Treatment Outcome in Comparison to a Waiting Phase." *Behaviour Research & Therapy* 43: 1,335–46.

Melzack, R. 1999. "From the Gate to the Neuromatrix." *Pain* (Suppl 6): S121–S126.

Miller, R. 2003. "Welcoming All That Is: Nonduality, Yoga Nidra, and the Play of Opposites in Psychotherapy." In J. J. Prendergast, P. Fenner, and S. Krystal (Eds) *The Sacred Mirror: Nondual Wisdom and Psychotherapy.* St. Paul, MN: Paragon House.

National Institute on Drug Abuse. 2018. "Opioid Overdose Crisis." Accessed May 14, 2018. https://www.drugabuse.gov/drugs-abuse/opioids/opioid-overdose-crisis.

Nisargadatta, M. 1985. *I Am That.* Durham, NC: Acorn Press.

O'Connor, P. J., and T. W. Puetz. 2005. "Chronic Physical Activity and Feelings of Energy and Fatigue." *Medicine & Science in Sports & Exercise* 37: 299–305.

Puetz, T. W., S. S. Flowers, and P. J. O'Connor. 2008. "A Randomized Controlled Trial of the Effect of Aerobic Exercise Training on Feelings of Energy and Fatigue in Sedentary Young Adults with Persistent Fatigue." *Psychotherapy and Psychosomatics* 77: 167–74. https://doi.org/10.1159/000116610.

Puetz, T. W., P. J. O'Connor, and R. K. Dishman. 2006. "Effects of Chronic Exercise on Feelings of Energy and Fatigue: A Quantitative Synthesis." *Psychological Bulletin* 132: 866–76. https://doi.org/10.1037/0033-2909.132.6.866.

Raub, J. A. 2002. "Psychophysiologic Effects of Hatha Yoga on Musculoskeletal and Cardiopulmonary Function: A Literature Review." *Journal of Alternative & Complementary Medicine* 8: 797–812.

Roelofs, J., G. van Breukelen, J. Sluiter, M. H. Frings-Dresen, M. Goossens, P. Thibault, K. Boersma, and J. W. Vlaeyen. 2011. "Norming of the Tampa Scale for Kinesiophobia Across Pain Diagnoses and Various Countries." *Pain* 152: 1,090–5.

Russell, I. J., P. J. Mease, T. R. Smith, D. K. Kajdasz, M. M. Wohlreich, M. J. Detke, D. J. Walker, A. S. Chappell, and L. M. Arnold. 2008. "Efficacy and Safety of Duloxetine for Treatment of Fibromyalgia in Patients with or without Major Depressive Disorder: Results from a 6-month, Randomized, Double-Blind, Placebo-Controlled, Fixed-Dose Trial." *Pain* 136: 432–44.

Smith, J. E., J. Richardson, C. Hoffman, and K. Pilkington. 2005. "Mindfulness-Based Stress Reduction as Supportive Therapy in Cancer Care: Systematic Review." *Journal of Advanced Nursing* 52: 315–27.

Stankovic, L. 2011. "Transforming Trauma: A Qualitative Feasibility Study of Integrative Restoration (iRest) Yoga Nidra on Combat-Related Post-Traumatic Stress Disorder." *International Journal of Yoga Therapy* 21(1): 23-37.

Streeter, C. C., T. H. Whitfield, L. Owen, T. Rein, S. K. Karri, A. Yakhkind, R. Perlmutter, A. Prescot, P. F. Renshaw, D. A. Ciraulo, and J. E. Jensen. 2010. "Effects of Yoga Versus Walking on

Mood, Anxiety, and Brain GABA Levels: A Randomized Controlled MRS Study." *Journal of Alternative & Complementary Medicine* 16: 1,145-1,152. https://doi.org/10.1089/acm.2010.0007.

Telles, S., B. R. Raghavendra, K. V. Naveen, N. K. Manjunath, S. Kumar, and P. Subramanya. 2013. "Changes in Autonomic Variables Following Two Meditative States Described in Yoga Texts." *Journal of Alternative & Complementary Medicine* 19: 35–42.

Telles, S., S. K. Reddy, and H. R. Nagendra. 2000. "Oxygen Consumption and Respiration Following Two Yoga Relaxation Techniques." *Applied Psychophysiology & Biofeedback* 25: 221–227.

Tolahunase, M., R. Sagar, and R. Dada. 2017. "Impact of Yoga and Meditation on Cellular Aging in Apparently Healthy Individuals: A Prospective, Open-Label Single-Arm Exploratory Study." *Oxidative Medicine and Cellular Longevity* 2017: 7928981. http://doi.org/10.1155/2017/7928981.

Tsang, A., M. von Korff, S. Lee, J. Alonso, E. Karam, M. C. Angermeyer, G. L. G. Borges, E. J. Bromet, G. de Girolamo, and R. de Graaf. 2008. "Common Chronic Pain Conditions in Developed and Developing Countries: Gender and Age Differences and Comorbidity with Depression-Anxiety Disorders." *The Journal of Pain* 9: 883–891.

Vachon-Presseau, E., M. V. Centeno, W. Ren, S. E. Berger, P. Tétreault, M. Ghantous, A. Baria, M. Farmer, M. N. Baliki, T. J. Schnitzer, and A. V. Apkarian. 2016. "The Emotional Brain as a Predictor and Amplifier of Chronic Pain." *Journal of Dental Research* 95: 605–612. https://doi.org/10.1177/0022034516638027.

Valdivia, B. S. 2014. *Reality Unveiled.* Google Books. https://play.google.com/books/reader?id=t6uoBAAAQBAJ&printsec=frontcover&pg=GBS.PP1

Van Houdenhove, B., and U. T. Egle. 2004. "Fibromyalgia: A Stress Disorder? Piecing the Biopsychosocial Puzzle together. *Psychotherapy & Psychosomatics* 73: 267–75.

Villemure, C., and M. C. Bushnell. 2002. "Cognitive Modulation of Pain: How Do Attention and Emotion Influence Pain Processing?" *Pain* 95: 195–9.

Violani, C., and C. Lombardo. 2003. "Peripheral Temperature Changes During Rest and Gender Differences in Thermal Biofeedback." *Journal of Psychosomatic Research* 54: 391–397.

Vollestad, J., M. B. Nielsen, and G. H. Nielsen. 2012. "Mindfulness- and Acceptance-Based Interventions for Anxiety Disorders: A Systematic Review and Meta-Analysis." *British Journal of Clinical Psychology* 51: 239–60.

Vowles, K. E., and L. M. McCracken. 2008. "Acceptance and Values-Based Action in Chronic Pain: A Study of Treatment Effectiveness and Process." *Journal of Consulting & Clinical Psychology* 76: 397–407.

Williams, K., C. Abildso, L. Steinberg, E. Doyle, B. Epstein, D. Smith, G. Hobbs, R. Gross, G. Kelley, and L. Cooper. 2009. "Evaluation of the Effectiveness and Efficacy of Iyengar Yoga Therapy on Chronic Low-Back Pain." *Spine* 34: 2,066–76.

Wood, C. 1993. "Mood Change and Perceptions of Vitality: A Comparison of the Effects of Relaxation, Visualization, and Yoga." *Journal of the Royal Society of Medicine* 86: 254–258.

Wood, P. B. 2010. "Variations in Brain Gray Matter Associated with Chronic Pain." *Current Rheumatology Reports* 12: 462–9. https://doi.org /10.1007/s11926-010-0129-7.

Wren, A. A., M. A. Wright, J. W. Carson, and F. J. Keefe. 2011. "Yoga for Persistent Pain: New Findings and Directions for an Ancient Practice." *Pain* 152: 477–480.

Yadav, R. K., D. Magan, N. Mehta, R. Sharma, and S. C. Mahapatra. 2012. "Efficacy of a Short-Term Yoga-Based Lifestyle Intervention in Reducing Stress and Inflammation: Preliminary Results." *Journal of Alternative & Complementary Medicine* 18: 662–7. http://doi.org/10.1089/acm.2011.0265.

Yurtkuran, M., A. Alp, and K. Dilek. 2007. "A Modified Yoga-Based Exercise Program in Hemodialysis Patients: A Randomized Controlled Study." *Complementary Therapies in Medicine* 15: 164–71.

Jim Carson, PhD, is a former yogic monk (swami) who has taught the practices and philosophy of yoga worldwide for more than forty-five years. Jim is now a clinical health psychologist; and associate professor of anesthesiology, and of psychiatry at Oregon Health and Science University (OHSU) in Portland, OR. He has applied his expertise to the development and evaluation of yoga and meditation-based clinical treatments, including the first mindfulness program for couples, the first loving-kindness meditation program for medical patients, and the Mindful Yoga program. Jim also works extensively with patients suffering from persistent pain, including those with fibromyalgia, low back pain, and cancer pain. Jim codirects national professional trainings for yoga teachers and allied health professionals at OHSU, Duke Integrative Medicine, and VA Centers. To learn more, visit www.mindful yogaworks.com.

Kimberly Carson, MPH, C-IAYT, is a mindfulness educator and yoga therapist at OHSU; specializing in the therapeutic use and scientific study of mindfulness and yoga for people with medical challenges. Kimberly currently offers mindfulness and yoga programs to chronic pain, cardiac, oncology (inpatient and outpatient), and internal medicine patients, and has taught mindfulness-based stress reduction (MBSR) for more than twenty years. In addition to codeveloping the Mindful Yoga program—which has been shown in research trials to significantly reduce pain, fatigue, and distress in those living with chronic pain—Kimberly consults on mindfulness and yoga clinical research trials, has coauthored dozens of peer-reviewed articles, and codirects professional trainings for yoga teachers and allied health professionals at OHSU, Duke Integrative Medicine, VA Centers, the Kripalu Center, and other locations around the country. With Carol Krucoff, Kimberly coauthored *Relax into Yoga for Seniors*. To learn more, visit www.mindfulyogaworks.com.

Carol Krucoff, C-IAYT, E-RYT, is a yoga therapist at Duke Integrative Medicine in Durham, NC; where she offers private sessions, workshops, and classes for people with health challenges. An award-winning journalist, Carol served as founding editor of *The Washington Post* Health section, and her articles have appeared in numerous national publications, including *The New York Times, Yoga Journal*, and *Reader's Digest*. She is author of several books, including *Yoga Sparks* and *Healing Yoga for Neck and Shoulder Pain*. She is codirector, with Kimberly Carson, of Yoga for Seniors Professional Training, and they are coauthors of the book (and DVD), *Relax into Yoga for Seniors*. She has served as a consultant on several yoga research studies, and coauthored articles in peer-reviewed medical journals. For more information, visit www.healingmoves.com.

MORE BOOKS *from*
NEW HARBINGER PUBLICATIONS

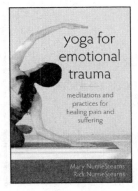
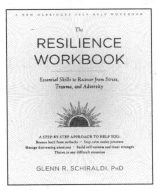
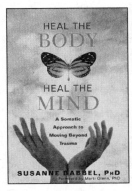
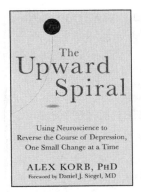
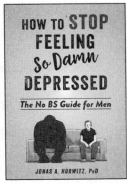
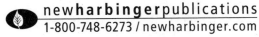

Register your **new harbinger** titles for additional benefits!

When you register your **new harbinger** title—purchased in any format, from any source—you get access to benefits like the following:

- Downloadable accessories like printable worksheets and extra content

- Instructional videos and audio files

- Information about updates, corrections, and new editions

Not every title has accessories, but we're adding new material all the time.

Access free accessories in 3 easy steps:

1. Sign in at NewHarbinger.com (or **register** to create an account).

2. Click on **register a book**. Search for your title and click the **register** button when it appears.

3. Click on the **book cover or title** to go to its details page. Click on **accessories** to view and access files.

That's all there is to it!

If you need help, visit:

NewHarbinger.com/accessories

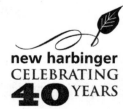

new harbinger
CELEBRATING
40 YEARS